Rob & Smith's

Operative Surgery

Genitourinary Surgery: Endoscopic Procedures
Fifth Edition

Rob & Smith's

Operative Surgery

General Editors

David C. Carter MD, FRCS(Ed), FRCS(Glas)
Regius Professor of Clinical Surgery, Royal Infirmary, Edinburgh, UK

R. C. G. Russell MS, FRCS
Consultant Surgeon, Middlesex Hospital and Royal National Throat, Nose and Ear Hospital, London, UK

Consulting Editor

Hugh Dudley CBE, ChM, FRCS(Ed), FRACS, FRCS
Emeritus Professor, St Mary's Hospital, London, UK

Art Editor

Gillian Lee FMAA, AIMI, AMI, RMIP
15 Little Plucketts Way, Buckhurst Hill, Essex, UK

Other volumes available in the series

Cardiac Surgery 4th Edition
Stuart W. Jamieson and Norman E. Shumway

The Ear 4th Edition
John C. Ballantyne and Andrew Morrison

General Principles, Breast and Extracranial Endocrines 4th Edition
Hugh Dudley and Walter J. Pories

Gynaecology and Obstetrics 4th Edition
J. M. Monaghan

The Hand 4th Edition
Rolfe Birch and Donal Brooks

Head and Neck 4th Edition
Ian A. McGregor and David J. Howard

Neurosurgery 4th Edition
Lindsay Symon, David G. T. Thomas and Kemp Clark

Nose and Throat 4th Edition
John C. Ballantyne and D. F. N. Harrison

Ophthalmic Surgery 4th Edition
Thomas A. Rice, Ronald G. Michels and Walter W. J. Stark

Orthopaedics 4th Edition
George Bentley and Robert B. Greer III

Paediatric Surgery 4th Edition
L. Spitz and H. Homewood Nixon

Plastic Surgery 4th Edition
T. L. Barclay and Desmond A. Kernahan

Thoracic Surgery 4th Edition
The late J. W. Jackson and D. K. C. Cooper

Trauma Surgery 4th Edition
Howard R. Champion, John V. Robbs and Donald D. Trunkey

Rob & Smith's

Operative Surgery

Genitourinary Surgery: Endoscopic Procedures

Fifth Edition

Edited by

Hugh N. Whitfield MA, MChir, FRCS
Consultant Urologist, St Bartholomew's Hospital and St Mark's Hospital for Diseases of the Colon and Rectum, London, UK

Butterworth–Heinemann
Oxford   London   Boston   Munich   New Delhi   Singapore   Sydney   Tokyo   Toronto   Wellington

Butterworth–Heinemann Ltd
Linacre House, Jordan Hill, Oxford OX2 8DP, UK

 PART OF REED INTERNATIONAL BOOKS

OXFORD   LONDON   BOSTON
MUNICH   NEW DELHI   SINGAPORE   SYDNEY
TOKYO   TORONTO   WELLINGTON

First published 1993

British Library Cataloguing in Publication Data
Rob & Smith's Operative Surgery. –
Genitourinary. – 3Vol. – 5Rev.ed
   I. Whitfield, Hugh N.
   617
   ISBN 0-7506-1240-1 (Endoscopic Procedures)
   ISBN 0-7506-1242-8 (3 volume set)

Library of Congress Cataloging-in-Publication Data
Rob & Smith's operative surgery. – 5th ed. / general editors, Hugh
   Dudley, David C. Carter, R.C.G. Russell.
       p.   cm.
   Includes bibliographical references and index.
   Contents: [1] Genitourinary.
   ISBN 0-7506-1240-1 (Endoscopic Procedures)
   ISBN 0-7506-1242-8 (3 volume set)
   1. Surgery, Operative. I. Rob, Charles. II. Smith of Marlow,
Rodney Smith, Baron, 1914–   . III. Dudley, Hugh A. F. (Hugh Arnold
Freeman) IV. Carter, David C. (David Craig) V. Russell, R. C. G.
VI. Title: Rob and Smith's operative surgery. VII. Title: Operative
surgery.
   [DNLM: 1. Surgery, Operative. WO 500 R6282]
   RD32R63   1993
   617′.91–dc20
   DNLM/DLC
   for Library of Congress   92-22884
                                                         CIP

Composition by Genesis Typesetting, Laser Quay, Rochester, Kent
Printed and bound in Hong Kong

Contributors

I. A. Aaronson MA, FRCS
Professor of Urology and Pediatrics and Director of Pediatric Urology, Medical University of South Carolina, 171 Ashley Avenue, Charleston, South Carolina, USA

D. H. Bagley MD
Department of Urology, Jefferson Medical College, Thomas Jefferson University, 1025 Walnut Street, Philadelphia, Pennsylvania 19107-5083, USA

A. J. Coleman MSc, PhD
Principal Physicist, Medical Physics Department, St Thomas' Hospital, London SE1 7EH, UK

M. J. Coptcoat ChM, FRCS
Consultant Urologist, King's College Hospital, Denmark Hill, London SE5 9RS, UK

R. C. L. Feneley MA, MChir, FRCS
Consultant Urologist, Southmead Hospital, Westbury-on-Trym, Bristol and Senior Clinical Lecturer, University of Bristol, UK

H. G. W. Frohmüller MD, MS, FACS
Professor and Chairman, Department of Urology, University of Würzburg Medical School, D-8700 Würzburg, Germany

M. A. Ghoneim MD
Professor of Urology, Urology and Nephrology Centre, Mansoura University, Mansoura, Egypt

L. G. Gomella MD
Department of Urology, Jefferson Medical College, Thomas Jefferson University, 1025 Walnut Street, Philadelphia, Pennsylvania, 19107-5083, USA

A. T. J. Holdoway BSc
Video South Ltd, 3 Kingsmead Square, Bath, Avon, UK

M. Kozminski MD
Phoenix Urology Institute, St Joseph, Missouri 64506, USA

J. McLoughlin MS, FRCS
Urological Registrar, Hammersmith Hospital, Du Cane Road, London W12 0HS, UK

E. Milroy FRCS
Consultant Urologist, The Middlesex Hospital, London W1N 8AA, UK

S. G. Mulholland MD
The Nathan Lewis Hatfield Professor and Chairman, Department of Urology, Jefferson Medical College, Thomas Jefferson University, 1025 Walnut Street, Philadelphia, Pennsylvania 19107-5083, USA

I. B. Nockler FRCR
Department of Radiology, St Bartholomew's Hospital, West Smithfield, London EC1A 7BE, UK

P. O'Boyle ChM, FRCS
Consultant Urologist, Musgrove Park Hospital, Taunton, Somerset TA1 5DA, UK

B. O'Donnell MCh, FRCS, FRCSI, FAAP(Hon)
Professor of Paediatric Surgery, Royal College of Surgeons in Ireland and Consultant Paediatric Surgeon, Our Lady's Hospital for Sick Children, Dublin 12, Ireland

K. F. Parsons FRCSEd, FRCS
Consultant Urological Surgeon, Royal Liverpool University Hospital NHS Trust, Prescot Street, Liverpool L7 8XP and Director of Urological Studies, University of Liverpool, UK

C. C. Schulman MD, PhD
Professor of Urology, University Clinics of Brussels, Erasme Hospital, 808 Route de Lennik, B-1070 Brussels, Belgium

P. J. R. Shaw FRCS
Senior Lecturer and Honorary Consultant Urologist, Institute of Urology, London and Consultant Urologist, St Peter's Hospital at The Middlesex Hospital, London and the Spinal Injuries Unit, Royal National Orthopaedic Hospital, Stanmore, Middlesex, UK

D. A. Tolley FRCS, FRCSEd
Director, Scottish Lithotripter Centre and Consultant Urological Surgeon, Western General Hospital, Edinburgh, UK

J. A. Vale FRCS
Department of Urology, St Bartholomew's Hospital, West Smithfield, London EC1A 7BE, UK

M. Vandenbossche MD
University Clinics of Brussels, Erasme Hospital, 808 Route de Lennik, B-1070 Brussels, Belgium

H. N. Whitfield MA, MChir, FRCS
Consultant Urologist, St Bartholomew's Hospital and St Mark's Hospital for Diseases of the Colon and Rectum, London, UK

G. Williams MS, FRCS
Consultant Urologist, Hammersmith Hospital, Du Cane Road, London W12 0HS and Honorary Senior Lecturer, Royal Postgraduate Medical School, London, UK

Contributing Medical Artists

Antoine Barnaud
11 Rue Jacques Dulud,
92200 Neuilly sur Seine, France

Joanna Cameron BA(Hons), MMAA
11 Pine Trees, Portsmouth Road,
Esher KT10 9JF, Surrey, UK

Peter Cox RDD, MMAA, AIMI
2 Frome Villas, Frenchay,
Bristol BS16 1LT, UK

Gillian Oliver MMAA, AIMI
15 Bramble Road, Hatfield,
Hertfordshire AL10 9RZ, UK

Richard Neave FMAA, AIMI
Unit of Art in Medicine,
Department of Cell and Structural Biology,
University of Manchester, Manchester M13 9PT, UK

Paul Richardson BA(Hons)
54 Wellington Road,
Orpington BR5 4AQ, Kent

Contents

Preface

Urological surgical practice is changing faster than any other branch of surgery. To some extent these changes have been promoted by a technological revolution, but others have occurred because of innovations in surgical techniques. The combination of this two-pronged strategy has made urology an exciting specialty to practise. But the rapidity of the changes has the disadvantage that both urological trainees and established urological surgeons have had difficulty in keeping abreast. There is also the necessity to recognize what changes have occurred for the better, which procedures will find a permanent place in the urological repertoire and which will come to be regarded as a passing fad.

This volume has been completely revised to take account of the changes which have occurred in the last 10 years. Greater emphasis has been placed on describing new techniques in detail, while more established procedures and those which have become less common are dealt with in less depth.

My thanks are due to many people who have helped to make this new edition come to fruition. The authors have given their time with good humour and great industry and to them I am indebted above all. My gratitude and admiration is also extended to the medical artists who have produced such a consistently high quality of illustrations, overseen by Gillian Lee. My thanks, too, to my secretary Alison Wrenn who has coordinated the activities of the authors, the publishers and myself with unfaltering patience. I am pleased to have been able to join forces again with David Carter, who was my mentor at an early stage in my surgical career, and with Chris Russell. Lastly, I would pay the greatest tribute to the patience and understanding of my wife Penny who has had much to endure during the preparation of this edition.

Hugh N. Whitfield

Illustrations by Peter Cox

Fundamentals of endoscope design

J. A. Vale FRCS
Department of Urology, St Bartholomew's Hospital, London, UK

History

There can be few fields of surgery in which minimally invasive techniques have made such a great impact as urology. In the early days of surgery, open operations on the bladder were frequently complicated by sepsis and urinary fistulae, whether performed via a transabdominal or transperineal approach. At the time of Samuel Pepys, bladder calculi were common and often treated by transperineal lithotomy, a procedure which was performed rapidly over 2 min with considerable morbidity and a mortality rate of almost 30%.

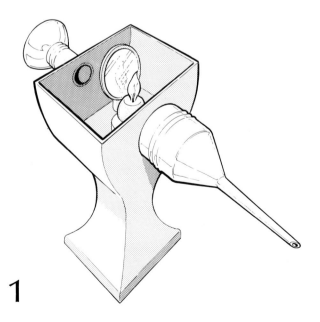

1 The greatest single advance in minimally invasive surgery was the development of the endoscope. Although attempts were made to visualize the inside of the bladder as long ago as Roman times, the first instrument recognizable as an endoscope was that developed by Phillippe Bozzini of Frankfurt between 1803 and 1808[1] (*Illustration 1*). It consisted of a simple silver tube which was illuminated proximally by a candle; the light from this was reflected down the tube by a mirror. Over the next 50 years numerous modifications were made to this basic design, but the instrument remained of little value due to its poor illumination. The claim made by Segalas[2] in 1826 that 'the light accumulated at the extremity of the urethral tube would enable a person to read the smallest printing type at a distance of 15 inches' must be regarded with some scepticism!

2 In 1853, Desormeaux[3] improved the illumination by replacing the candle with a lamp powered by a mixture of turpentine and alcohol, but the field of view remained no greater than the tube diameter. It was 1879 before this problem was overcome, with the production of the Nitze–Leiter endoscope (*Illustration 2*). This was the first endoscope to resemble a modern rigid cystoscope and incorporated all three essential components of a modern rigid system: distal illumination, a lens system and an instrument channel. This was improved further with the invention of the Edison bulb in 1891, which replaced the rather cumbersome platinum wire light source that had been used in the original Nitze–Leiter cystoscope.

There were numerous modifications to cystoscope design in the first half of the 20th century, including the Amici prism to correct image inversion and the introduction of prisms to achieve an angled field of vision. However, the greatest milestone was the introduction of fibreoptics in the 1950s. Fibreoptics can be defined as the propagation of light along thin fibres of transparent material by multiple total internal reflections (MTIR). Interestingly, the phenomenon of MTIR had been elegantly demonstrated to the Royal Society by John Tyndall in 1870: he showed that light could be guided along a curved jet of water. The potential significance of this was not realized until the 1950s when the technology was available to produce tiny flexible glass fibres. Professor Harold Hopkins at Reading University introduced the first clad glass fibre in 1951[4], and in 1957 Hirschowitz[5] passed the first prototype gastroscope down his own gullet. Since then the science of fibreoptics has progressed rapidly, particularly with respect to the upper gastrointestinal tract, and by the early 1970s rigid gastroscopes had become largely obsolete. Advances included the incorporation of channels for suction and irrigation to keep the objective lens clear, and the development of a deflectable tip. The development of flexible fibreoptic instruments for the urinary tract has been slower, probably because modern rigid urological instruments

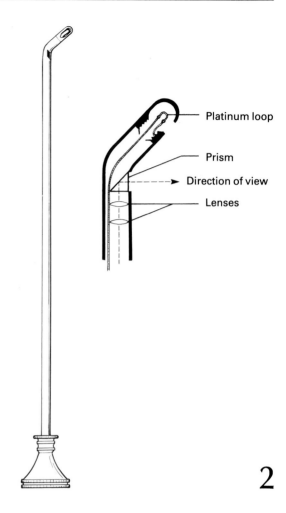

Platinum loop

Prism

Direction of view

Lenses

2

are so satisfactory and can reach most sites for which they are required – for example, the entire ureter can be negotiated with a rigid ureteroscope. However, it is important to remember that fibreoptic technology is used to transmit the light to the tip of a modern rigid instrument from an external light source, so replacing the need for a bulb at the objective end of the telescope. It seems ironic to reflect upon the similarities between this arrangement and that used on the very first endoscope designed nearly 200 years ago by Bozzini, where once again the light source was external to the patient!

3a, b

Although the introduction of fibreoptics was undoubtedly a major milestone, it was not the only great advance of the 1950s. Hopkins transformed the optics on rigid telescopes by introducing a rod lens system in 1956[6]. Older cystoscopes had a series of field and relay lenses separated by long air spaces (*Illustration 3a*). Although the lenses were designed to keep as much light as possible within the endoscope, there were inevitable losses as some rays hit the telescope casing. The latter had to be rifled to suppress reflection of this stray light, and this reduced the light aperture for a given external telescope diameter. The rod lens system (*Illustration 3b*) overcomes these problems, permitting a greater clear aperture for a given telescope diameter and improving light transmission.

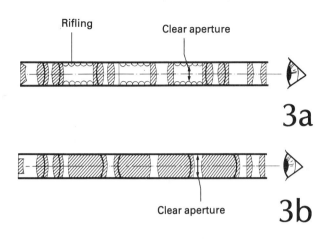

Rigid endoscopes

Contemporary rigid endoscopes incorporate three essential features: a rod lens system, a fibreoptic bundle for transmission of light from an external source to the bladder, and an irrigating channel to flush away blood and dilate the organ under vision.

Rod lens system

4

This is the optical system of the telescope, and comprises an objective lens to create a real and inverted image of the object at I_O and a series of rod lenses to relay this image to I_E. The eyepiece lens has an action similar to that of a simple magnifying glass, and produces a magnified virtual image at I_V. As the image is inverted at each relay, the number of rod lenses is selected to ensure that the final image is erect.

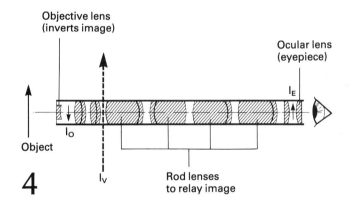

5 The high quality of modern optics has enabled instrument manufacturers to produce objective lenses with a wide range of viewing angles. The viewing angle is the angle formed by the two outer limits of the telescopic image and determines the field of view. The usual viewing angle is 60–70°, but larger angles of over 100° can be generated using 'fish eye' lenses. This can expedite orientation and inspection, but at the expense of magnification and definition peripherally.

Many telescopes contain reflecting prisms just behind the objective lens to deviate the optical axis to the desired direction of view. The direction of view represents the relationship of the optical system to the horizontal axis of the telescope, and is also the middle of the viewing angle. The directions of view that are commonly available in cystoscopes are 70°, 30° or 12° (the so-called foroblique angle) and 0°, which requires no prism. The 70° telescope is ideal for obtaining a panoramic view, while the 30° and 12° scopes are usually used for manipulation – for example transurethral resection. Prisms produce single-axis inversion of an image, and therefore a second 'K' prism is always necessary to reinvert the image at the eyepiece. Telescopes without a prism (0°) are useful for negotiating passages such as the urethra, although foroblique telescopes can be used in this situation.

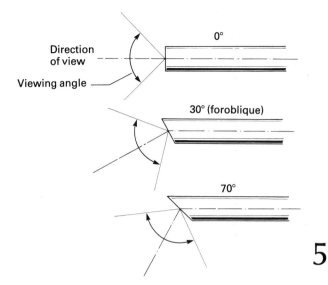

5

Fibreoptic bundle

This is the means of light transmission to the objective end of the telescope, and runs down the periphery of the telescope. As the light bundle is not concerned with image transmission, it is made from incoherent fibres and is relatively cheap to produce. At the objective end of the bundle is a lens to ensure even distribution of light over the field of vision, and the bundle is angulated to coincide with the visual angle of the instrument. At the eyepiece of the telescope the bundle terminates as the light pillar, to which the light bundle from the light source connects.

Irrigation/instrument channel

6, 7 This may be an integral part of the endoscope, as in a typical nephroscope (*Illustration 6*), or contained within a sheath into which the endoscope fits (*Illustration 7*). The latter is the arrangement commonly used on cystoscopes, the telescope locking into the sheath by means of a 'bridge'. This provides a watertight locking system, and may contain also a catheterizing port for introducing ureteric catheters or manipulative instruments such as biopsy forceps.

Two types of irrigation systems are available: intermittent irrigation in which the irrigant enters and is emptied via the same lumen, and continuous flow. In the latter, irrigating fluid enters by an inner channel while it is sucked out simultaneously through an outer sheath. The advantage of this system is that the urologist can perform a procedure such as transurethral resection of the prostate without stopping repeatedly to evacuate the bladder. This can be particularly useful when performing a prostatectomy on a low-capacity bladder such as may develop secondary to long-term infravesical obstruction.

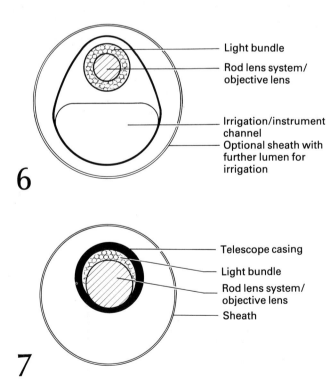

Physics of fibreoptics

8 As mentioned earlier, fibreoptics can be defined as the propagation of light along thin fibres of transparent material by multiple total internal reflection (MTIR). For this to occur, the transparent fibre must be enclosed by a material of lower refractive index such as air or a different type of glass. The phenomenon is explained by considering the processes of refraction and reflection at the boundary between the two materials. The lower medium is glass with a refractive index n_g and the upper medium may be either air or glass with a lower refractive index n_a. A ray of light travelling through the lower medium and hitting the boundary surface at point P with incident angle A (*Illustration 8a*) will be refracted and travel through the upper transparent medium at the angle B; it is therefore lost. The relationship between the angles A and B is given by the equation:

$$n_g \sin A = n_a \sin B.$$

As the angle of incidence A is increased, the angle of the refracted ray B also increases according to the above relationship. When A equals A_c (the 'critical angle' of incidence), the refracted ray will travel along the boundary surface (*Illustration 8b*). The critical angle for any two substances will exist when angle $B = 90°$ ($\sin B = 1$), and therefore the critical angle A_c is determined by the equation:

$$\sin A_c = n_a/n_g.$$

If the angle of incidence is increased beyond this critical angle, the ray is totally reflected at the boundary surface (*Illustration 8c*). It is this condition of total internal reflection that enables glass fibres to transmit light. Rays that strike the boundary at angles of incidence less than the critical angle will be lost, and there is therefore a 'maximum acceptance angle of incidence' for light transmission. This is not determined solely by the critical angle, as it must allow also for refraction occurring at the point of light entry into the fibre.

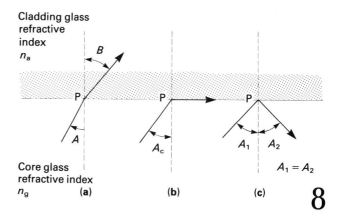

Cladding glass refractive index n_a

Core glass refractive index n_g

(a)   (b)   (c)   **8**

9 There are two types of fibreoptic bundle within a flexible endoscope, one concerned with image generation and the other with light transmission into the body. To create an image using fibreoptics, a large number of fibres need to be grouped together. The pattern formed by the colour and intensity of the individual fibres is perceived by the observer as an image. For the image at the eyepiece to duplicate the image at the objective end of the bundle, it is essential that the ends of each individual fibre occupy the same relative position at both ends of the bundle. This is a so-called 'coherent' bundle or image-guide bundle.

For MTIR to occur, each glass fibre bundle must be enclosed by a material with a lower refractive index than the core glass; in practice this fibre cladding is usually glass with a different composition. The resolution of a particular image-guide bundle will depend upon the diameter of the fibre core, the thickness of this cladding, and the alignment and orderliness of the packing of the fibres at the ends of the bundles. The ratio of the total area occupied by the individual fibre cores to the total area of the fibre bundle is referred to as the 'packing fraction'. As it is only the cores which transmit the image, the ideal image-guide bundle should have a high packing fraction and yet multiple very small fibres to provide good resolution. In reality the final product is a compromise: cladding cannot be less than 1.5 μm thick, and if the fibres are made too small the high proportion of cladding area within a bundle will result in a very dark image. The smallest practical fibre diameter is limited to about 8 μm, which relates to a packing fraction of 60%.

Fibre bundles used for light transmission are referred to as light-guide bundles. There is no need for ordered arrangement of fibres relative to each other, and these bundles are referred to as 'incoherent'. Furthermore, resolution is not an issue and the individual fibres are made much thicker (30–50 μm) permitting a bigger packing fraction and more efficient light transmission.

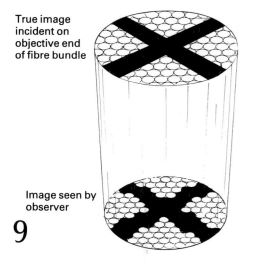

True image incident on objective end of fibre bundle

Image seen by observer

9

Manufacture of fibreoptics

High-precision well-ordered coherent fibre bundles are extremely difficult and time-consuming to produce. The two main production methods are the leaching method and the rotating-drum technique. In the former, the initial fibre starts out as a single glass rod consisting of a core of high-quality optical glass, a cladding of glass with a lower refractive index and a second cladding of acid-leachable glass. This original rod has a diameter many times greater than that of the final fibre. The necessary number of these rods (usually more than 25 000) are perfectly aligned within a large cylinder of acid-leachable glass. This master image-guide is then placed in an electric furnace and pulled until the individual fibres are reduced to the desired size of approximately 8–10 μm.

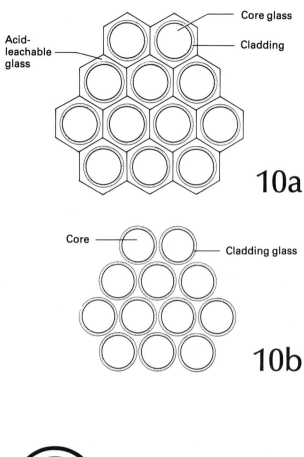

10a, b During the heating and pulling process, the acid-leachable glass is forced into a hexagonal honeycomb pattern (*Illustration 10a*) and the fibres become fused as a single rigid bundle. In order to confer flexibility on the bundle, which is dependent on the very fine fibres moving freely relative to each other, the ends of the bundle are fixed in protective holders and the bundle is soaked in acid. The acid-leachable glass is dissolved, leaving a bundle in which the ends are fixed but the fibres are otherwise free and flexible (*Illustration 10b*). Thus a high-quality flexible bundle has been produced while protection of the ends has guaranteed that the bundle is coherent.

11 In the rotating drum method of manufacture, a single very long (perhaps 75 km) fibre is carefully wound around a rotating drum in the manner of a reel of cotton. The fibres are then clamped together at the top of the drum, and the sides of the drum removed. The clamp is sawn in half with a diamond saw and the two ends polished.

The manufacture of light-guide bundles is very much simpler, as the fibres have a larger diameter and the bundle is incoherent. Needless to say, this is reflected in the price: it costs about £100 to produce a light guide compared with £1500 for an image guide.

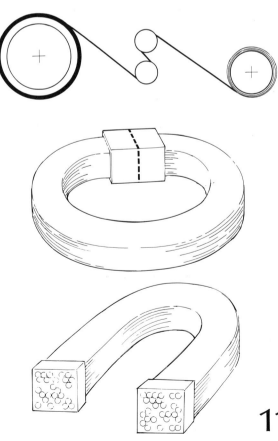

Flexible endoscopes

12 The main components of a flexible endoscope include the optical system, the illumination system, a bending section/angulation system and an irrigation channel. These are all contained within an outer insertion tube.

Optical system

13 This comprises the image guide (IG), together with lenses at the objective end and eyepiece of the endoscope. The objective lens forms an image of the object under view (X_o) on the distal face of the image guide (X_d). Light representing this image is transmitted through the image guide and a duplicate image is formed on the proximal face of the bundle (X_p) at the eyepiece. As the objective lens produces an inverted image on the distal face of the bundle, the image on the proximal end of the bundle (X_p) will also be inverted; this is overcome by having a 180° twist in the image guide. The eyepiece contains an ocular lens that serves as a simple magnifying glass, producing an enlarged virtual image (X_v) of the tiny image at the bundle tip.

Illumination system

This consists of the light guide, and special lens systems at both ends of the bundle to capture the maximum amount of light from the light source at one end, and produce a wide angle of even illumination at the other.

Bending section and angulation system

One of the advantages of a flexible endoscope over a rigid one is the ability to angulate its tip to obtain a wider field of vision, and perhaps to negotiate a narrow orifice such as the neck of a bladder diverticulum. To achieve this, the flexible scope needs an angulation system and a bending section. The latter is constructed of a series of interlocking metal rings, the pivot points permitting controlled movement of the rings on each other. Flexible cystoscopes are usually designed to flex in two directions, with a total arc of about 250°; one arc is at least 160°, permitting the telescope to look back on itself and provide an excellent view of the bladder neck. It is possible to design endoscopes that can flex in any direction by alternating the pivot points on the metal rings by 90°; this arrangement is used on the standard gastroscope. Angulation is achieved by means of wires running down the length of the insertion tube, and attached to a control knob via a chain and sprocket within the control section of the endoscope.

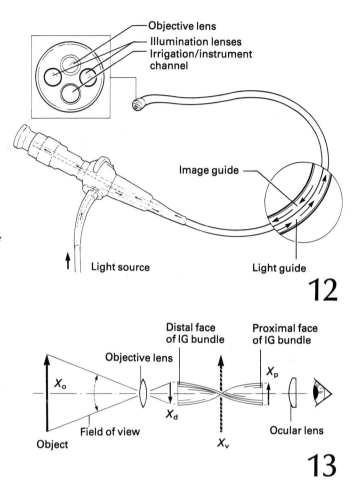

Objective lens
Illumination lenses
Irrigation/instrument channel

Image guide

Light source

Light guide

12

Distal face of IG bundle

Proximal face of IG bundle

Objective lens

X_o

X_d

X_p

Field of view

Object

X_v

Ocular lens

13

Irrigation channel

This is simply a channel running the length of the telescope, which can be used for irrigation and the passage of flexible instruments such as biopsy forceps.

Insertion tube

This is constructed in three layers. The inner layer comprises helical steel bands, which give the endoscope its circular cross-section and protect it against compressive forces. There is then a thin layer of stainless steel wire mesh, covered on its outer surface by a plastic sheath. These layers prevent the endoscope from twisting and stretching, and the plastic protects it from the corrosive action of some disinfectants. Most modern instruments are completely watertight, thus facilitating 'cold' sterilization by immersion in glutaraldehyde or iodophor disinfectants.

Light sources

A variety of light sources are available, ranging from low-power simple halogen sources to sophisticated xenon units. A powerful xenon unit is essential if a teaching aid or videocamera is attached, as these accessories result in an enormous loss of light; the beam-splitter in a standard teaching attachment steals 80% of the light to service the secondary image guide.

High-intensity light sources generate intense heat, and dichroic coatings and heat-absorbing filters are essential to filter out this non-visible radiation; these are usually sited within the light unit itself.

The future

At present there can be little doubt that, where access permits, the rigid endoscope is preferable to its flexible counterpart. For any given external diameter, a rod lens system will offer three times the resolution and superior channels for irrigation and insertion of accessories[7]. This is largely because of the space occupied by the intricate metal skeleton and angulation systems on the flexible endoscope. The small flexible instrument channel permits only the use of small flexible graspers and forceps, which are often working at such gross mechanical disadvantage that they are ineffectual. Thus the role of the flexible endoscope has been a primarily diagnostic one. However, this situation is changing with the development of laser technology and electro-hydraulic devices for stone disintegration: these probes can be less than 1 mm in diameter.

As with so many advances of the late 20th century, microchips may provide the technology for the ultimate endoscope. In the 'video optic', all optical elements are replaced by a microchip sensor and electrical wiring; the image is electronically generated and displayed on a screen. As yet the system is expensive and largely experimental, but perhaps in 200 years' time urologists will regard our current technologies in much the same way as we regard the candle and mirror of Bozzini!

References

1. Edmonson JM. History of the instruments for gastrointestinal endoscopy. *Gastrointest Endosc* 1991; 37: s27–s56.

2. Editorial. Description of an instrument for inspecting the urethra and bladder. *Lancet* 1826–7; ii: 603–4.

3. Desormeaux MAS. De l'endoscope, instrument propre a éclairer certaines cavités intensely de l'économie. *C R Acad Sci* 1855; 40: 692–3.

4. Hopkins HH, Kapany NS. A flexible fibrescope using static scanning. *Nature* 1954; 173: 39–41.

5. Hirschowitz BI, Curtiss LE, Peters CW, Pollard HM. Demonstration of a new gastroscope, the 'fiberscope'. *Gastroenterology* 1958; 35: 50–3.

6. Hopkins HH. Optical principles of endoscopy. In: Berci G, ed. *Endoscopy*. New York: Appleton Century Crofts, 1976: 3–63.

7. Miller RA. Endoscopic instrumentation: evolution, physical principles and clinical aspects. *Br Med Bull* 1986; 42: 223–5.

Cameras for endoscopy

Alistair T. J. Holdoway BSc
Video South Ltd, Bath, Avon, UK

The solid-state imaging chip has now replaced the camera tube as the basis for colour television cameras in most fields. The device that has become standard is referred to as a 'CCD', or charge-coupled device. The CCD has revolutionized television cameras in a very short time and presents many advantages to the manufacturer of specialist cameras for endoscopy: these include the reduced size and weight, low power consumption, improved safety, improved image quality and higher reliability. This has led to a greater awareness of the advantages of using television in endoscopy and a greater interest in the design of units to meet such specialist demand. It is worth noting, however, that in common with so many other high technology devices, the development of the basic electronics is so expensive that it is unlikely that a single company would design any specialist camera in total. The reality of this situation is that the very large manufacturers design and produce a variety of cameras that they hope will have wide appeal in general applications such as security surveillance or television programme making; specialist manufacturers then use the core electronics to build a camera suitable for specialist application. The skill of the specialist manufacturer is to recognize those attributes of a television camera that are important in his market place and then to choose the 'base camera', from a large producer, that has the best existing mix of benefits in electronic performance and features. He must then design in as many other features as the specialist market requires. Some of these will be electronic modifications and some will be ergonomic and physical features.

In the design of a camera for urological endoscopy, a number of desirable features not available from any manufacturer of 'base cameras' can be listed: these include such attributes as a soakable head and cable, a high safety standard, an easy-to-use plug on the camera cable, a camera socket on a controller fitted to the front of the unit, and infrared filter for use with lasers, etc. The low-volume production of these cameras and the frequent update in the design of special features account for both the high price and the sometimes less than acceptable reliability, when compared with those of the off the shelf units from which they are derived. The other fact arising from this manufacturing process is that comparing the essential characteristics of various cameras is usually inconclusive. The image quality defined by resolution, colour definition and sensitivity is governed by the 'base camera' design and, at any one time, most designers of endoscopic cameras are aware of the leaders in these specifications and will change their base camera at short notice to keep up with picture quality. When comparing the latest models from a wide range of makers there is usually little difference in basic performance (with exceptions – usually indicated by price). A more worthwhile assessment of an endoscopic camera is of the features particular to the application, especially those which relate to ease of use, long-term reliability and safety. These are more difficult parameters to satisfy in the operating theatre environment and these factors have more impact on manufacturers' costs than do the basic image quality parameters that are defined by the 'base camera'.

Background

Image sensors

The image sensor now used in the design of colour television cameras for endoscopy is the CCD. *Figure 1* shows how such chips are arranged. The light-sensitive surface has a regular pattern of picture elements or 'pixels'. When light falls on these pixels a transfer of electrical charge related to light intensity takes place. These points of electrical charge are then measured at the output in a time-related way, via a shift register, and this is interpreted as a television picture. The output of the shift register is very different in nature to a scanned output from a picture tube and gives a measure of voltage related to time that allows viewing or recording equipment to reconstruct the same image.

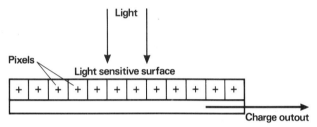

Figure 1 Simplified cross-section of a charge-coupled device (CCD)

Three types of CCD design are available. *Figure 2* shows diagrammatic representations of the 'full-frame read', 'frame transfer' and 'interline transfer' CCDs. The full-frame read is the smallest type but, as it does not have a storage register in which to 'dump' the charge pattern while another image is being created, the illumination must be removed while the image is scanned out. Although this is all happening in very short time periods (1/50–1/1000 s), the absence of light for up to 50% of the operating time makes the sensitivity poor. The frame transfer design offers the best combination of sensitivity and resolution. The imaging surface is always available to light and the resultant charges are periodically dumped into the storage register and then 'scanned out' from the horizontal shift register. This design is seldom used in miniature cameras because it is the largest type of CCD. The interline transfer CCD has a storage register that is integral with the picture elements, such that each pixel is actually an image cell and a storage cell. This reduces the resolution and sensitivity but the benefits in size and lack of streaking from highlights (a problem with early CCDs) make this the choice of most manufacturers. It is now possible to make this type of CCD with over 400 000 pixels, which gives a resolution adequate for most endoscopic viewing.

This so far describes only how a CCD can capture a monochrome image. There are two ways to produce a colour image: the one used by high-quality television

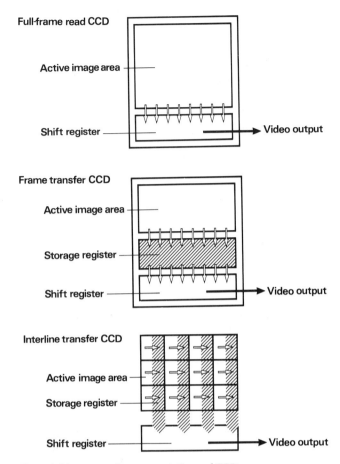

Figure 2 Diagrammatic representations of CCDs

cameras (broadcast) is to use three CCDs, to split the incoming images into their red, green and blue elements and to focus these separated images on individual sensors; the other method (*see Figure 3*) is to superimpose a mosaic filter so that each pixel is also giving information on the percentage of colour in that area. By scanning out the charge from each pixel in a time-related way, the value of luminance (the basic image detail) and chrominance (the percentage values of red, green and blue) at each point of the image sensor surface is known. The choice of colours and quality of the mosaic filter will have a significant effect upon the crispness and colour fidelity of the resulting image.

Cy	G	Cy	G	Cy	G	Cy	G	Cy
Y	G	Y	G	Y	G	Y	G	Y
Cy	G	Cy	G	Cy	G	Cy	G	Cy
G	Y	G	Y	G	Y	G	Y	G
G	Cy	G	Cy	G	Cy	G	Cy	G

Figure 3 Mosaic filter based on cyan, green and yellow

PAL format

Once collected, the image has to be conveyed to other devices for the purpose of viewing or storage. There is a great deal of detail in a colour television image and moving images are conveyed at a rate of 25 complete frames per second. To accommodate this very large amount of information a large bandwidth of frequencies is required and several ways of achieving this have been developed. Different basic signal standards are used worldwide (PAL, NTSC and SECAM) and there are also different ways of conveying television signals within those standards.

There are three main television standards to which equipment can conform. In the UK and most of Europe the PAL standard prevails; in France and Russia SECAM is used but such is the prevalence of PAL equipment in neighbouring countries that most non-broadcast equipment is now PAL; in the USA and Japan, NTSC is the standard. A comparison of these standards would be a text in itself but in a world where goods are easily bought and sold over territories it is important to know that NTSC will only work with NTSC and PAL will only work with PAL. There are so many differences between the two standards that changing the signal from one type to the other can only be accomplished with some very exotic hardware. Luckily for the Europeans, PAL is a later development (1967) of colour television and is superior in colour fidelity. The only disadvantage of a PAL environment is that, as most basic television technology is developed in the USA and Japan, the very latest cameras are usually available in NTSC first.

It is a great advantage to the television user that the local standard is rigidly adhered to. Unlike computers, any television camera will work with any video recorder and any monitor. The only exceptions to this are where a manufacturer has 'cheated' on the rules (not unknown in endoscopy) or if the equipment, although being PAL, is conveying the signal in a different way.

Television waveform

Television images are conveyed from one device to another in an analogue waveform. This high frequency, wide bandwidth and complex waveform must be preserved in all recordings and connections if image quality is to be maintained. It is circuitry of wide bandwidth and high stability that has always separated high quality television from other electronics, in price if not in complexity. *Figure 4* is a composite waveform showing the basic essentials of a television signal. The bandwidth of such a signal could be up to 5.5 MHz and contain as much information as up to 2.5 megabytes every 25th of a second if digitized! As shown on this waveform, there are important features that are not in the picture area, in particular the 'line synchronization pulse' and the colour burst. These are two critical features which if badly generated (by poor camera

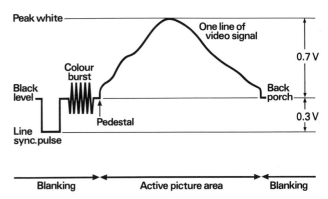

Figure 4 Television signal waveform

circuitry) or distorted in recording will cause major image disturbance or colour loss. As these features are not 'seen' it is sometimes the case that poor cameras will work on a local monitor (the most tolerant device in television) but for seemingly unexplained reasons the recorded or transmitted images are almost unusable. Unlike digital computer signals, television deteriorates significantly each time the signal is recorded or conveyed in any way and, in common with all analogue waveforms, it is the precision of the original signal that has the key part to play in maintaining quality in a correctly configured system.

Single- or multi-chip cameras

In order to achieve a colour television picture, the earliest cameras were equipped with four imaging tubes – one for luminance and one for each of the primary colours (red, green and blue). This was reduced to three tubes when it was discovered that the luminance information could be taken from the green channel. Three-tube cameras have remained the standard broadcast configuration, until very recently when CCD technology reached the resolution of tubes. In the early 1970s the colour single tube was developed by putting a filter with extremely fine stripes of blue and red on the tube. By scanning such an arrangement it was possible to define mathematically the red, green, blue and luminance at each point on the imaging tube face. Resolution was, at first, poor and colour a little soft and single-tube cameras never attained a quality adequate for broadcast or serious programme makers; however, they were common in medicine for all uses, including microscopy and endoscopy.

When the CCD first emerged, many believed that a single-chip device could be developed with sufficient resolution and colour fidelity (without the scanning problems of an electron beam) to avoid a return to multi-element cameras. This did not prove to be the case and soon 3-CCD cameras were designed with an optical block, similar to the tube predecessor, splitting the image into red, green and blue components.

Because each CCD in this arrangement is working in monochrome, maximum resolution and colour quality can be achieved. The drawbacks are that some light sensitivity is lost in splitting the image to each chip and the optical block can be reduced only to a finite size and weight. Another solution has been tried by a major manufacturer using two chips, one for luminance and one for chrominance; this solution has not yet been widely accepted.

The majority of endoscopic cameras are single chip. For most users the increased image quality of a three-chip camera is outweighed by the small size, light weight and lower cost of a single-chip camera. In terms of the image quality, a single-chip camera can now produce up to 400 lines resolution whereas a three-chip camera can produce 750 lines.

Performance of a camera

The 'base camera' chosen by the endoscopic camera manufacturer defines most of the image quality characteristics. The desirable attributes of such a base camera are the same as those required by other camera users, as outlined below.

Resolution
This describes the ability to resolve black on white lines in the horizontal plane. For a good single-chip camera this is about 350 and for a good three-chip this is about 700. It should be noted that this resolution is directly related to the available bandwidth and, therefore, all other devices in the system through which the signal passes will critically affect resolution. For instance, a standard VHS recorder has a bandwidth that allows a resolution of only about 230 lines.

Sensitivity
This is complicated by the technique for measurement. Variables include monochrome or colour subject, speed of the lens, and agreed value at which the output is too low; this value may include the use of gain control (electronic amplification) in the camera control unit. Sensitivity is very important in endoscopy where underexposed images at the limit of illumination are common. However, the figures quoted in specifications are difficult to interpret or compare.

Signal-to-noise ratio
This is a ratio measured in 'db' for 'noise' occurring in the picture. Noise in a television signal manifests as a background pattern of 'snow' effect, which has the result of diminishing perceived resolution and colour quality.

Dynamic range
This is not a widely accepted measurement for television cameras and is seldom quoted. However, in endoscopy this could be a very useful value to compare as it is the difference between the lightest and darkest features in a scene that can be visualized adequately. This is particularly relevant to achieving a 'good distance view' endoscopically, when tissue close to the endoscope tip is highly illuminated and the far view is much more weakly lit. This is also true in the bladder, where the size of the cavity disperses the available light and yet direct views of mucosa are overexposed.

Camera design for endoscopic urology

Ergonomic characteristics

A camera to be attached to either a rigid telescope or a small fibrescope is preferably as small and as light as technology will allow. As always, there is compromise because the smallest and lightest CCD camera that an engineer can design may lack other attributes that are either vital or highly desirable. The key factors affecting size are the optical mount, the camera cable attachment and the soakable design.

Optical mount
For a camera of maximum versatility, a 'C' mount thread for optics is the choice. A wide range of couplers for every make of endoscope is available in this standard. Beamsplitters and direct couplers of a variety of focal lengths can be fitted to the camera at any time. Adaptors are also available for all makes of microscope and an enormous range of lenses are based on this mount, which has been common since early cinematography days. If a camera is to be shared between departments, then this is a highly desirable feature. The penalty for a 'C' mount is that it is 25 mm in diameter and this limits miniaturization.

Camera cable attachment
The camera cable should also be as light and flexible as possible, while having the required strength for constant use in the operating field. All microchip cameras have a complex multicore cable and attaching this securely to the camera head with its many almost microscopic connections to the CCD chip is a design problem. The easiest way to satisfy the immediate physical problem of durability is to mount the chip in a very small body, with the cable already fixed, and then to fill the entire body to the rear of the chip with high quality plastic, which is also moulded out along the cable for a short way to give adequate strain relief. This

will give a very strong, watertight and permanent connection of the smallest possible size. The penalty for this method is that if the camera cable should be damaged anywhere from its midpoint to the camera, then as it will be impossible to replace the cable, an entire new camera head will be the only solution to one of the simplest reasons (and certainly the most common) for failure of an endoscopic video system.

A more common solution is to house the chip in the smallest possible complete case and to create a traditional cable gland to the rear of the chip, through which the cable passes and is clamped. The cable ends are then attached to the circuit board upon which the chip is mounted. The cable gland must be waterproof and provide a length of strain relief up the cable. This necessitates the gland being manufactured from relatively soft plastic and being glued or moulded to the cable. This method places a lower limit on size and allows repair of the camera or replacement of the cable at the factory. When the camera cable fails, the camera will be out of service for several weeks and the cost of a quite complex repair will be high.

Some camera manufacturers recognize that reliability and low down-time are eventually seen by any market as high priority and they have designed soakable cameras with a plug and socket at the camera head. This entails the CCD chip being mounted in a complete housing with connections available for a plug. The plug has to be a sealed unit with high quality connectors and a good seal to the camera head, and with a gland for strain relief of the cable. The space taken up by mounting a socket on the camera head, and a suitable plug coupled with waterproof seals, means that the plug and socket almost double the size of the camera head. The advantage to the user is that when the camera cable breaks it can be changed locally in minutes. This prevents frustrating down-time and lowers replacement costs to the cost of the cable itself; in the area of high-technology electronics, labour costs are very much greater than those of spare parts.

Soakability

A camera for urological endoscopy must be soaked and the disinfectant most commonly in use is based on glutaraldehyde. Although some users have decided that soaking the camera before each procedure is not warranted, nevertheless it will become very wet in routine use and will need thorough cleaning and disinfecting on a regular basis. These disinfectants are highly corrosive and also leave residue, if not carefully washed off. It is therefore necessary for all parts of the camera, cable and plug to be sealed, easy to clean and made from resistant materials.

A good design ensures that even the plug that connects to the camera control unit meets this specification, because the camera and cable are much more easily handled and cleaned if all parts are soakable and can be treated as sterile when required. The plugs of

this design are not a traditional multipin, but are a specially developed high quality 'edge connector' with rare-metal plating and a tough moulded body; this design is easy to check and to keep clean.

Traditional plug designs used on some cameras are usually fitted with an end cap to seal them when soaked. This seldom works well in practice, as it would be unusual to test such items routinely, but they are likely to leak eventually. The fitting of a cap whenever the camera or cable could get wet leaves room for significant human error. A traditional multipin round plug will deteriorate quite quickly when exposed to even the slightest moisture on a regular basis; it is impossible to clean or dry between the pins, should this become necessary.

Optical characteristics

It is necessary here to distinguish between the camera itself and optics that are fitted to it. This is not always as easy as it sounds, as specialist manufacturers may make the two inseparable, or entirely modular, or any intermediate combination. The camera is the electronic part of the assembly. This is a miniature camera head containing the imaging chip and with a cable to the camera control unit (which contains all the other processing electronics and is not just a power supply) that is an integral part of the camera. Within the camera may be fitted filters appropriate for the type of lighting to be used. In front of this is an optical coupler which performs several functions – focuses the image on to the chip, gives any image magnification required (or determines how much of the image is seen by the chip), and connects the camera physically to the endoscope. Many styles of coupler exist, with free rotation or locking and with quick release or not: a direct coupler allows only the camera to have a view from the endoscope; a beamsplitter allows the operator to see into the end of the endoscope and the camera to have a view. Generally, direct couplers are in a straight configuration between the camera and the endoscope, whereas beamsplitters position the camera at right angles to the endoscope.

An interesting development in urology and gynaecology is that most surgeons using a camera for resection use a beamsplitter, even though they view only directly from the television screen. The reason for this is that the right-angle position of the camera is both comfortable for the operator and also helps him to maintain 'life' orientation on the screen by ensuring that the camera is always hanging down but allowing the endoscope eyepiece to rotate freely; this gives an orientation that is easy to control. If the camera is allowed to move with the endoscope while resecting, then normal orientation is lost, which is disconcerting.

These optics conform to various basic types of mount which currently fall into four types. The so-called 'glass mount' is the smallest possible arrangement in which the camera is mounted directly to the glass end of the telescope, which has a removable eyepiece or no eyepiece; usually such a camera can be used only with the endoscope for which it was designed. The 'V' mount was developed by American manufacturers as a small-diameter standard; a limited range of direct couplers and beamsplitters are available. The 'C' mount is the best established mount, with a wide range of optics available. Some cameras are made with an integral direct coupler; these were largely designed for arthroscopy and this design can be very limiting in other fields.

The filters that could be usefully fitted to all endoscopic cameras include an absolute cut infrared which assists when neodymium yttrium aluminium garnet (NdYAG) lasers are in use and a crystal filter which helps reduce moiré patterning, which can be a problem when using any type of fibrescope.

Electronic characteristics

Cameras built for endoscopy consist of a miniature camera head and a camera control unit (CCU); only the two units together can be referred to as a complete camera. In an ideal world, all the circuit boards would be packaged with the imaging chip in a single 'camera body'; however, as the basic technology is produced by very large general manufacturers, various electronic features must be added or modified by the endoscopic camera designer to suit the application. The six features that have proved most important in practice are the colour bar generator, the white balance, automatic light-level control, choice of outputs, multiple camera heads, and function button.

Colour bar generator

When this is switched on, it replaces the camera image with a recognizable pattern of vertical stripes of white, yellow, cyan, magenta, red, green, blue and black. This very dependable output is useful to check that the whole video system is working, even if the camera is not connected (e.g. while it is soaking) and is vital if the camera seems to produce no image, in which case the colour bar is a known good signal to test all the other equipment. The signal can also be recorded or printed and proves that these devices are working well in every colour. Without this facility, loss of picture due to failure of any component will remain undiagnosed.

White balance

With many cameras now being operated with more than one type of light source, it is necessary to have a guaranteed way of resetting the colorimetry of the camera. The two main types of light source in use are halogen and xenon. The colour output of a lamp is measured as colour temperature in degrees kelvin. A halogen lamp gives a 'warm', rather yellow light and is actually the standard on which cameras are measured in the factory at a colour temperature of 3200 K. These lamps are fitted in the familiar 150 W endoscopic low-power light sources. Xenon lamps are much more powerful, at over 300 W, but produce a very cold blue light of about 6000 K. These are popular with urologists using television, as the power is necessary for good imaging in the bladder, especially with a 70-degree telescope. The effect of different colour temperature illumination on a television camera is very much greater than it is to the eye, which makes such corrections quite quickly. The white balance control allows the camera to correct for this very different lighting. Setting the white balance is usually done by pointing the endoscope, with camera attached, at a white swab (or similar non-reflective white surface) and, with the image correctly exposed, the white balance control is pressed. This not only improves overall hue, but also colour separation and therefore perceived clarity of the image. It is useful if a manual hue control is provided to make subsequent minor adjustments to colour.

Automatic light-level control

For some time, light sources have been available that automatically adjust their output to expose the camera correctly; they do this by feeding the camera signal to the light source and reacting to the total signal level (which should be 1 V at optimum). However, there are two reasons why this does not work well: one is that an endoscopist moves the telescope quite fast most of the time and the light source cannot be made to react quickly enough; the result of light level 'following' the requirement is that it works against the intention. The second reason is that although an evenly illuminated screen should produce a signal of 1 V (this is a general television standard), the typical endoscopy view is not evenly illuminated and the information required could be in a poorly illuminated part of the image. If the light source adjusts to cope with any flare, then darker portions will go black. It is more effective to use a constant illumination and to move the endoscope to achieve correct exposure.

A different way of achieving automatic exposure is more appealing: the CCD chip can be made to 'expose' electronically and subsequently to unload its image at varying rates; at higher speeds the exposure time is lower. The latest technology allows the camera to measure its own output on different parts of the chip and then to compensate by raising or lowering this rate and therefore the exposure. This system allows the light source to be left at one setting and for the camera to react very quickly to correct exposure.

Choice of outputs

The various types of signal format to convey the camera image to other devices are discussed above. With the range of equipment now available that may be incorporated in a system, all cameras should have one or, better still, two composite video outputs. This is the most common signal to feed monitors, video recorders, printers, etc. An S-VHS [or Y/C (luminance/chrominance)] output should be provided for use with a growing number of high quality video recorders and monitors that require this. For the very serious user an RGB (red, green, blue) output will give the highest possible quality on a suitable monitor and is also necessary for good results on the latest video 'still frame' technology, such as disc recorders or printers.

Multiple camera heads

This facility is possible only on some cameras: not all cameras can match extra camera heads to one CCU. This facility can be useful in a very busy department that depends on television imaging, or when a system is shared between departments. The camera head and cable account for at least 80% of breakdowns in video systems and a spare could be useful.

Function button

Even though camera heads are now very small, some manufacturers have been able to incorporate a button on the camera head. This facility allows the surgeon to control remotely another device in the system which could be the start/stop on a video recorder, the print command on a video printer, or any other device that the system designer can interface to a simple switch.

Solving practical problems

Diathermy interference

A longstanding problem of using cameras in operative endoscopy is the potential for interference from electrosurgical equipment. For the urologist resecting prostates and bladder tumours, this can be a very frustrating problem. There is, to date, no perfect solution or complete theory to enable an interference-free image to be obtained for any combination of diathermy and camera. It has become clear, however, that the interference is picked up by the camera in three main ways and from this a systematic approach to mitigating the effect has been developed.

It should be noted that some combinations of diathermy and camera do not interfere at all, but even these are complicated by some individual (and unexplained) exceptions. Electrosurgical generators are, by their nature, high-power, high-frequency devices. These high frequencies fall within the video bandwidth and can cause major picture disturbance. The three main ways in which the camera picks up this interference are mains-borne, air-borne and conducted.

Mains-borne interference

This occurs when the diathermy passes high frequencies back down the mains cable and these are picked up by the mains supply to the camera. This can be reduced to a minimum by fitting a filter to the mains input to the diathermy (available from the manufacturer) and by connecting the camera to a mains supply as far away as possible from the diathermy. This problem is also greatly aggravated by poor mains wiring (especially earthing) within the hospital.

Air-borne interference

The diathermy emits a range of high frequencies in radio bandwidth. The camera cannot be totally shielded in metal because the CCD must be able to 'see'; radio waves can always reach it, therefore, and are also induced into cables and circuit boards. This is a very difficult problem if the generator frequencies are close to the main operating frequencies of the camera (and many are). Two ways in which this radiation has been successfully limited are by connecting a filter on the diathermy cable at the connection to the generator and by carefully limiting the output of the generator to a power only just high enough for effective cutting.

Conducted interference

This interference can be generated at the diathermy unit or separately by the arc between the cutting instrument used and tissue. A certain size of arc is necessary for smooth and successful cutting and the arc itself is a spark generator, creating a wide range of frequencies and especially harmonics of the diathermy output. Coagulation mode which is pulsed bursts of high frequency and can also produce such effects from the pulsing frequency as well as from the main output frequency. As the patient forms part of the diathermy circuit and the endoscope is within the patient, it is reasonable to assume that such radio interference can be induced into the metal parts of the endoscope, the camera and probably the surgeon too (weakly).

Avoidance of interference

It is difficult to differentiate between air-borne and conducted interference but some practical measures can be taken to keep these to a minimum. A power setting no higher than is necessary to achieve a good cut or coagulation, and disposable pads using electrolyte gel, seem to reduce this type of interference; the precise position of the pads on the patient also seems important. Some experiments have also suggested that the arc can be kept to a minimum for good cutting by developing a feedback circuit for diathermy generators. This measures the amplitude of harmonics produced by the arc and adjusts the output power very rapidly to keep them at a preset level as cutting proceeds. As yet, this theory has achieved no practical success; it is to be hoped that cooperation between camera manufacturers and diathermy manufacturers will 'design out' this irritating problem.

Obtaining a high-quality image

Any two endoscopic cameras produced in the same year by two reputable companies will have a very similar specification for picture quality. The reasons why some systems seem to produce superb results whereas others look mediocre, are factors other than the performance of the camera. When the image on the television screen is too poor to use and yet the direct view down the endoscope is reasonable, the response is often to blame the new advanced technology, yet this is almost certainly not culpable, as a CCD camera is only an imaging chip with processing electronics; this technology tends to be either working perfectly or to have a major problem. A weak or unsuitable picture with poor clarity and colour will not be attributable to the camera (in 90% of cases) because neither the CCD or other parts of the circuit tend to suffer from slow deterioration of drift. The most likely causes of a poor image are: (1) condensation between the optical coupler and the eyepiece of the endoscope; (2) moisture seeping between the optical coupler and the camera (if it is removable) or moisture leaking into the optical coupler itself; (3) the quality of the endoscope – a slightly inferior endoscope that seems in excellent condition on visual inspection, can produce, nevertheless, a very indistinct television image. Regularly used endoscopes suffer from abrasion at the distal tip, causing microscopic scratches that create very cloudy effects. Soaking in disinfectant and not rinsing thoroughly will cause a build-up of residues, which become almost opaque. Slight flexing of the endoscope causes light-guide fibres to break and reduces the light output at the tip. Irrigation is also an important factor: slight cloudiness of the irrigant fluid does not have too adverse an effect on the eye but has a very marked effect on a camera. When using a television camera it is best to use either an irrigating resectoscope or to wash out much more regularly.

It is the optical quality of the image presented to the CCD that governs image quality. Good endoscopes, good optical couplers, clear irrigant and a high-power light source, all meticulously checked, will produce the best results.

System design

As well as the camera, other features of the system are very important to allow easy use of television, and they also have an effect on the final image: these features are described in detail in the chapter on pp. 19–26. Television cameras have now reached such a high level of quality and ease of use that viewing the procedure from a monitor is now feasible and has many benefits for the urologist.

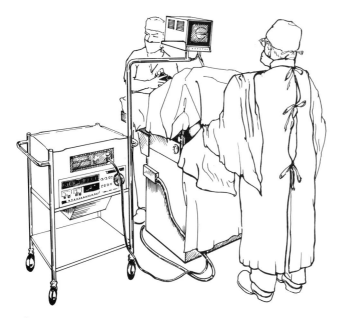

1 The ideal design of a system for a urologist will incorporate an easy way to position the monitor screen directly in front of the surgeon over the table. It is important that the viewing monitor is of a high quality and safe specification: television sets should never be used in an operating theatre. When evaluating a complete system for urology it is necessary to ensure that the camera outputs match the monitor that is desirable, the video recorder required and any device such as a printer. It may also be necessary to consider whether the signal is to be fed to any other monitors in theatre or in a room nearby, or perhaps to a teleconference system in a teaching area.

1

Future prospects

The technology of video imaging has been improving very rapidly. Cameras will continue to give better images within existing standards and will be refined for endoscopic use by becoming smaller and more automated. Soon, all cameras will have a good automatic exposure and will set up automatically for the different colour temperature of light sources; this leaves the surgeon with no user controls at all. It is also likely that a new generation of endoscopes based entirely on fibres that run from the endoscope tip to the CCU/light source will emerge. In this arrangement a light source is incorporated in the CCU, as is the CCD imaging chip. The optical fibre can be up to 2 m long and carries light and image. The fibre can be fitted to an endoscope that has no other optical parts, but which carries out all the required physical functions. The advantage of such a system is that there are less constraints on the size of the imaging chip assembly and two major costs are avoided – the design of a soakable camera head and the necessity of having several telescopes. The disadvantage is that the quality of rigid telescopes is very hard to match and at present it is difficult to make such fibres with various angles of view. Other designs will include a camera built on to the endoscope instead of an eyepiece and, if CCDs can be made sufficiently small, an electronic endoscope without optics but with the CCD mounted on the distal end.

Developments in television will be especially valuable in high-quality still-image capture and in the next 5 years digital recording methods will be available that will greatly enhance editing, archiving and 'transport' of images. High-resolution television, which has been in the pipeline for over 5 years already, will emerge when the politics of worldwide television allow. This new television standard allows an intrinsic doubling of potential resolution and the resulting images are very much more useful for documenting. However, introduction is not governed by technical constraints, but by major interests in broadcasting for the next century. Certainly, any equipment produced in the first 2 or 3 years of such development will be prohibitively expensive.

Video systems for endoscopy

Alistair T. J. Holdoway BSc
Video South Ltd, Bath, Avon, UK

The simplest video system for an endoscopist consists only of a camera and a viewing monitor. Indeed, some manufacturers, who wish to present the most user-friendly unit possible, have incorporated the camera controls into a monitor housing and thereby have integrated the basic components. Most camera designers, however, retain the established format of a camera control unit with outputs to a monitor and other devices; this is the more flexible approach, but flexibility brings choices.

As well as a viewing monitor, there is a range of equipment that might usefully be connected to the camera in the operating theatre: this includes video tape recorders, video printers, still frame recorders, video typewriters and, perhaps, further monitors. It may also be desirable to connect the camera with equipment outside the theatre, for demonstrations or central documenting. Incorporating all this potential facility into an easy-to-use and reliable video system for use in theatre demands electronic and ergonomic design with the endoscopist's environment in mind.

Background

The camera

The detail of camera design and the facilities available are dealt with in the chapter on 'Cameras for endoscopy', pp. 9–17. When considering a camera in a system more complicated than connection only to a monitor, various facilities may be important. If the total system is to be shared between two or more disciplines, then a range of optical adaptors may have to be supplied to fit a range of endoscopes. The most adaptable cameras are fitted with a 'C' mount. For these cameras, optics are available to fit them to all endoscopes and all microscopes, as well as standard lenses. If the camera is to be used in only one department, then a more restricted optical arrangement may suffice. Electronically, it should be noted whether a camera has the correct signal outputs for connection to other video components of the system. All cameras sold in Europe should conform to the PAL standard for recording and transmission in order to operate with all other equipment. There are four different types of output in use, within the standard, for connecting cameras to various other devices: these are composite (the most common), S-VHS, RGB (red, green, blue) and component; the latter is a broadcast format and is not used except with cameras of high specification (usually three-chip). The other three are found in any combination on various cameras. The implications of having each of these outputs are as follows.

Composite

All cameras should have this output. Until 1989 it was quite unlikely that any other type of output would have been offered and it remains the most common way to connect video equipment. The single coaxial cable carries the entire vision signal and all equipment using this format is entirely compatible.

S-VHS [or Y/C (luminance/chrominance)]

This is an increasingly useful output to have on a camera. A growing range of equipment is configured for this format and it has allowed higher-quality images to be achieved from smaller and less expensive equipment. The S-VHS recording format bears little relation to the original VHS system except in mechanics. The very high image quality is suitable for copying and editing, but demands the use of a Y/C signal throughout the system. Thus, a range of equipment all based on Y/C is now available, including recorders, monitors, edit suites, mixers, etc. Many pieces of such equipment are now provided with composite and Y/C inputs and outputs. If the camera has a Y/C output then it is a good idea to use this and configure the system with other components that use it. In particular, it seems that the emerging video still-frame recording and printing devices work well in Y/C mode.

RGB

This is a signal format that has been used in studios for many years and is now becoming more and more popular for technical applications. Most high resolution monitors will accept RGB signals and produce crisper images with higher colour fidelity when connected in this way. This is also a common standard with which to connect cameras to computer inputs for graphic creation or image analysis. A variety of new technology for the recording and reproduction of still images is also best used in RGB mode; however, this is not a signal used by video tape recorders, standard television mixing or switching equipment. Any camera with an RGB output should, therefore, also have a composite output to feed standard devices while the RGB is used for primary monitor and for specialist documentation. The four coaxial wires (usually individual) used for interconnection by RGB have also sometimes limited the use of this format in non-studio applications.

Deciding on a particular system to suit a purpose and provide a range of facilities is therefore best done by defining the facilities required, listing the general type of equipment in the system to perform these tasks and then selecting items that operate well together, including a camera which is also comfortable to use. The average system used by a urologist in theatre will consist of an endoscopic camera, one or two monitors, a video tape recorder and possibly a video printer for hard-copy images. Some systems are also equipped with video caption generators to enter patient details and time/date to a recorded image.

Video monitors

Domestic television sets should never be used in an operating theatre or connected to an endoscopic camera. Televisions are not sufficiently safe or durable and do not have facilities suitable for this purpose. Good-quality video monitors are justifiably more expensive and a very wide range is available. The most common sizes are 9, 14, 20, or 28 inches, from most manufacturers.

1   For the urologist, a 9-inch can now be the most convenient primary viewing monitor. It is possible to design video system trolleys that can hold a small monitor over the operating table directly in front of the surgeon. This size monitor can be 12-V powered, which is necessary for safety in the operating field. The 12-V transformer powering this unit can be fully isolated and protected with a very low-leakage current. Some pioneers in this field of video prostatectomy used Mayo tables or platforms fixed to the table to support the monitor, but this has the distinct disadvantage that the monitor must still be connected to the rest of the system for video signal and power. A mobile system with a movable arm to position the monitor over the table with integrated cables is preferable.

Another way to achieve this is to mount the monitor on a ceiling arm. This has the advantage of allowing even more flexible positioning on a rotating arm, which is countersprung. It is now possible to feed the low voltage and the video signal through the slip-rings in such an arm, to allow absolute freedom of rotation with no visible wires. These small monitors are designed for high-quality applications and give a very sharp and intense image. The proximity to the eye gives a very coordinated feel to using the television system for direct viewing. In this arrangement it is common to have a secondary monitor to enable other theatre staff to view the procedure: this is usually a 14-inch on the system trolley or a 21-inch mounted on the wall; 28-inch monitors are usually mounted on walls in larger theatres or in adjacent seminar rooms or rest areas. When choosing particular monitors for an operating theatre system, the following points should be noted.

First, the primary monitor should be positioned for ease of use by the surgeon. No other facilities are necessary, but it must produce the highest-quality image that the camera is able to provide and must be safe to use in all respects. Connecting a high-quality camera to a mediocre monitor effectively links the two pieces into one set of electronics and degrades the output.

Second, the secondary monitor may be of lower image quality (except when part of a documenting system) but may need more facilities: these may include audio if the system is fitted with a video recorder, NTSC and PAL display if the system is fitted with a video recorder that has the capability to play back American

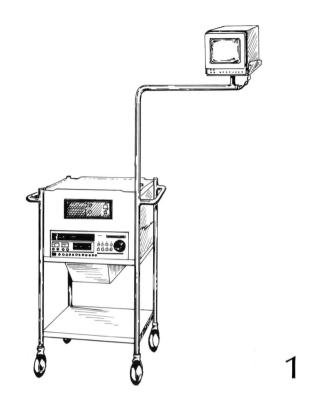

1

recorded tapes, a variety of inputs to monitor images from different devices in the system, and video/audio outputs if the signals may need to be 'looped' to further monitors. If several monitors are to be linked to the output of the camera or video recorder, then it may be desirable to fit a distribution amplifier to the system, to split and amplify the signal into several outputs of equivalent level and quality.

Video tape recorders

There are currently eight video cassette recorder (VCR) formats that are used in hospitals: these are 8 mm, high band 8 mm, VHS, Super-VHS, U-Matic, high band U-Matic, Betacam SP and M11. This represents a wide range of quality, facility and price. Betacam and M11 recorders are approximately 50 times as expensive as an 8 mm or VHS domestic recorder. Choosing from this vast range of equipment to suit a system depends upon two main considerations: the first should be the intended use of the recordings, and the second should be whether a particular machine of the type required meets the specification for reliability and ease of use. As well as these two factors there may be choices between individual machines, based on useful facilities.

Consideration of what will be done with the recordings will immediately limit the possible choices. If recordings are to be reviewed only on the video system in a local seminar room, then VHS or 8 mm may be adequate. These formats were designed down to a price for home use and have very limited resolution and colour fidelity. If recordings are merely for review, then the ability to replay almost anywhere on inexpensive machines and from small cassettes with long record time can be convenient. However, neither of these formats can be used when any copying or editing is envisaged. Video tape editing is a sophisticated way of duplicating the required sequences of an original tape on to a new tape. If editing will be required to create compilations or programmes for conferences or teaching, then a tape standard for which good editing equipment is available, and which duplicates well, is necessary. These qualifications do not yet apply to high band 8 mm which, although significantly better quality than 8 mm, does not have full editing available.

Super-VHS and U-Matic are the standards most commonly used by hospital departments in the UK. U-Matic has now been available for 16 years and is therefore the longest-running video format available. Furthermore, this format has always been upwardly compatible: that is, all tapes recorded on previous machines will play on later models. The latest quality is high band SP and despite the fact that the method of recording the signal has changed a great deal, it is still possible to replay tapes recorded on standard U-Matic built 16 years ago. Many hospitals have U-Matic edit suites available as a shared facility and, where this is so, this is a sensible machine to use if editing and copying for non-broadcast programmes is envisaged. Super-VHS is a newer format (introduced 1989) which has a quality similar to U-Matic but with some differences. The main difference is that to achieve full S-VHS quality the VCR must be fed with a high-quality Y/C signal and, in turn, must feed a monitor with a Y/C input. When S-VHS machines are used with composite feeds, then much of the extended potential quality is lost. S-VHS machines must also be used with special S-VHS tape; if standard VHS tape is used, then the electronics automatically default to standard VHS mode. VHS/S-VHS is upwardly compatible: normal domestic VHS prerecorded cassettes will play on S-VHS recorders. However, S-VHS tapes will not play on a normal VHS recorder. Therefore, recording S-VHS in order to have acceptable copy quality is no more flexible than any other format, as there are not likely to be other S-VHS recorders at home or elsewhere for casual playback. More and more hospitals are installing S-VHS edit suites because the cassettes are much smaller than U-Matic and are available in up to 3-h rather than 1-h lengths.

Betacam and M11 are broadcast cassette formats that will be used more and more in teaching and training applications, as there are now several even higher-grade broadcast formats. These machines use derivatives of Beta and VHS cassettes, respectively. However, the recording method bears no relation to domestic video equipment. These machines can record a much greater bandwidth and use a much higher writing speed to achieve this. The edit capabilities and copy quality are very high, and most broadcast television programming has been originated in these formats between 1982 and 1991. Both Betacam and M11 can record from composite signals but the best possible quality is achieved when they are fed with component or Y/C. There are probably few hospitals (perhaps four or five at present) with editing at this level. However, if recordings are to be made into high-quality programmes for broadcast, conferencing by satellite or for mass duplication to standard VHS copies, then these high original standards must be used. If the final tape needs to be copied to NTSC for use in quantity in America or Japan, or sent by satellite, then such a quality of edited tape is also mandatory. It is likely that more and more departments that participate in distance learning will invest in this type of equipment, which will probably become relatively less expensive as even higher-quality formats begin to be used in broadcast.

Having decided which format is demanded by the applications for video recording, the second main consideration of suitability must be investigated. The attributes of a video recorder of value when being built into a system for operative endoscopy are as follows:

1. High build quality, robust to the harsh environment of the operating theatre which can often be very humid, warm and has a corrosive atmosphere, is necessary. Use by many different staff also produces high wear and tear.
2. A suitable remote stop/start control obviates the need to ask staff to do this; the control could be a function button on the camera head or a foot control.
3. A 'real-time' clock counter allows an accurate record to be kept of the location of recordings of interest on any one tape. This count is from the tape and is repeatable on edit suites, thus allowing recording notes to be made to assist another person to locate specific excerpts.
4. Two independent audio channels with microphone inputs on the front of the machine will ensure easy recording of audio both in theatre and as a voice dub. If video tapes are to be used for any type of presentation, then a sound-track of good quality recording in the theatre is invaluable. The spontaneous commentary is often more useful than a subsequently recorded 'voice over' and, even if a programme is to be made with a carefully edited voice track, the background sound effects from theatre and occasional use of the spontaneous voice brings life into the programme. For tapes intended only for use in the department, the regular use of a microphone enables 'note taking' at the time of operation, which can be invaluable in confirming details on review. With two independent channels, the amateur producer can always record a track in theatre and then dub a voice over on to the second track without altering the first; there is then a future choice as to which track is played, or they can be mixed.

Video stills

Video still-imaging devices will emerge in the 1990s as an important part of endoscopic video systems. As more and more endoscopists of all types are working from the television screen, there is a demand to create high-quality 'photographs' from the video camera image rather than periodically exchanging the video camera for a photographic camera for the purpose of creating hard copy. Indeed, technical factors in both the endoscopy field and in photography are also creating a pressure in this direction. Endoscope manufacturers are looking for ways by which to create the completely electronic endoscope that gives a video signal as an output but has no optical channel, and photographic equipment manufacturers, who have to satisfy the consumer market to remain competitive, are producing cameras of less flexibility and adaptability for techniques involving specialist optics. The high-quality video still (when it arrives) will solve many current problems of film, including ease of use (what you see is what you get) and storage. The advantages in the latter area are common whenever electronic media take over: still images can be stored electronically in very much smaller formats and can also be entered automatically into a database at the time of creating the image. This logging and library keeping allows images to be searched for in a variety of ways, just like any other relational database, and can ensure that images are permanently coded with relevant details so that they are never confused or lost. Still-imaging hardware will include magnetic discs that store 50–100 images (useful to replace the photographic camera at point of work). The images chosen can subsequently be printed or loaded on to a larger file, on analogue optical discs which will store up to 72 000 images. This system preserves the highest image quality and the machines are operated under computer control as part of a database and can be displayed with computer data inserted. Digital disc stores as part of computer hardware are currently storing up to 40 images on a disc (these images have to be digitized first, some quality is lost thereby, but once stored they can be transferred between computers many times). Video printers of various sizes are now available to produce hard copy in a photographic print format or on transparency for overhead projection. Send and receive workstations can now allow high-quality video stills to be sent by audio wire or telephone line over any distance to allow communication. This range of hardware has, at present, two missing components: these are a good technique for making slides, and an inexpensive magnetic disc on which images can be stored and either kept with notes or taken to a central facility for printing or storage on a larger database. The latter is very close to introduction, but high-quality slides from a video source are difficult to produce and at present the equipment is either much too expensive or unsatisfactory in performance. Of course, the magnetic disc will allow easy projection, using large-screen video, but this is not suitable for international conferences or book publishing.

Designing a system

Endoscopy system in theatre

The key attributes of a video system to be used by a urologist day by day are ease of use, reliability and safety. These are of greater concern than the peak-of-image quality or a wide range of functions or accessories that are seldom used. These attributes apply not only to each individual piece of equipment in the system but also to the design of the overall package. It is possible to have a very good camera, video recorder, monitor and other hardware which, in themselves, are quite satisfactory by these measures but which, when put together in a working system, are either physically clumsy, electronically badly matched or just too complicated to use when all put together.

A fundamentally good design should package the equipment together to produce the least number of separate, free-standing pieces of equipment linked by wires. For a very simple system comprising a camera and a monitor, some companies have already incorporated the camera controls in the monitor housing, leaving only one cable to the camera. This is a good concept for a very simple unit. Most urologists carrying out transurethral resections now prefer to work directly from the monitor to improve comfort when operating. To do this effectively requires a design of a monitor mounting over the patient directly in front of the surgeon. This can be done in several ways, but the most effective is usually to hold the monitor on a movable boom arm fixed to a trolley in which the other video equipment is housed (see Illustration 1). If the 'over the table' monitor is not an integral part of the complete video system (for instance if it is put on a Mayo table or clamped to the table), then cables carrying power and video must link it to the other equipment. This is not very easy to use and can be quite dangerous when equipment or patients are moved in and out of theatre. The monitor being fixed to an arm on a substantial mobile trolley means that the whole system, with integral cables to the monitor, can be wheeled about in the theatre without risk. In the body of the trolley (which must be of a certain minimum size and weight to perform this task) can be housed such other equipment as is required. This can include instruments for video recording, video printing, time and date generating (to insert on video recordings or prints), caption generating and the camera control unit. The trolley can also hold a second monitor (pointing away from the surgeon) for staff and students to view and also the high-power light source (still a necessity, especially for bladder work). Such a trolley should be as enclosed as possible, with the equipment fixed. This has several advantages: mains

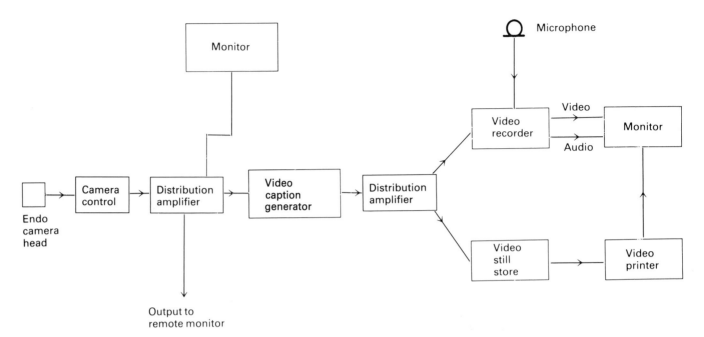

Figure 1 System diagram for an endoscopic video system with full facilities

distribution can be internal to the trolley and separately fused or even isolated, and the equipment is more secure and tamper-proof. The equipment is better protected from accidents (fluid spills, etc.) and with all the interconnecting wiring enclosed it is likely to be more reliable over a longer period. An aspect of safety that is important for the over-table monitor is that it should be powered by low voltage from a high-quality transformer. It is not satisfactory to place a 240-V monitor over a patient and close to the surgeon, especially as there may be many connectors at the monitor. Low-voltage monitors are available; it is therefore necessary for a transformer to be built into the trolley. Finally, the trolley can also be equipped with a drawer to house the smaller loose items, such as the camera head, optics, microphone and accessories.

The total equipment in a package will depend upon the facilities that an individual finds useful. *Figure 1* is a block diagram of what could currently be described as a full-facility system comprising (1) camera and camera control unit; (2) caption generator for patient details inserted to the video image; (3) over-table monitor; (4) monitor on trolley top (14-inch) with audio; (5) video tape recorder with clip-on microphone; (6) video printer for hard copy; (7) video still-image recorder for recording individual stills of each patient for later printing or loading to a database; and (8) video distribution amplifier, to give enough video outputs from the camera. In some larger operating theatres it may also be desirable to connect an output from the system on a larger monitor mounted on the wall, so that all other staff may comfortably view procedures.

Systems outside the operating theatre

It is becoming more common for those involved in teaching to transmit images out of the theatre to a remote location. In the simplest form this could just be an output from the endoscopic camera fed to a monitor in a local seminar room or rest area. If the system is equipped with a microphone, then audio could also be fed to the remote monitor. If it is envisaged that meetings could be conducted with small groups in this way, then return sound could also be provided to enable the audience to comment back to the surgeon.

More sophisticated systems that allow comprehensive presentations to be made to remote audiences are now becoming more common, as teaching modern endoscopic techniques can now be carried out entirely by television and with views superior to those obtained by being in the theatre. To teach in this way it is necessary to allow the audience to have more than just an endoscopic view and a commentary: it is also necessary for an expert audience to have a view of the theatre showing layout, patient preparation, nursing procedures and technical equipment. A view from over the surgeon's head or shoulder is desirable in order to demonstrate the precise operation of equipment, as well as external anatomy and manipulations. Any imaging equipment such as radiographic or ultrasonographic machinery used in theatre will also produce vital information that must be fed to the viewer. Thus, a video system capable of full presentation for teaching urology to a remote audience would ideally have the following elements: (1) a good-quality endoscopic video system; (2) a video camera mounted high on a wall giving a good 'plan' view (this would preferably have remote controlled pan/tilt and zoom lens); (3) a video camera mounted on an arm of the theatre lamp assembly to give views of open procedures and 'over shoulder' shots; (4) a link from any ultrasonographic or radiographic machinery; (5) a miniature clip-on microphone for the surgeon to use; (6) an extra microphone for others to comment to the audience; (7) an easy-to-use console that allows selection of the video image that the audience is viewing, controls for the cameras and the two-way audio equipment. This is quite an array of equipment. However, electronics of this type have become a great deal smaller and if such equipment avoids a crowded theatre and enables teleconferences to be carried out, then it is certainly worthwhile.

The teleconference system described above allows the medical staff in an operating theatre to send the audience one of any four specific views at any one time, with sound commentary from the surgeon and one other, and with the ability of the audience to talk back. Such a system should also be equipped with an 'off-air' intercom to allow the audience chairman to talk to the theatre (and vice versa) in private for the purpose of setting up schedules or discussing timings, and also if there is a technical fault in the teleconference system that requires consultation. With such a system in place, the audience can be located in a room anywhere in the hospital grounds and can watch in comfort either on a large monitor or on a large-screen projector. The latter is becoming the usual viewing device in lecture rooms designed to hold over 50 persons. The quality is now excellent and pictures can be projected on to white screens or walls of sizes from 48 to 200 inches diagonal. Live presentations have a great deal more impact when shown on large screen and the life-size appearance of the operating theatre imparts a much greater degree of reality to the audience.

Editing and archiving

The difficulty about regularly recording procedures in theatre is having a good system to access the required excerpts when they are required. Many hours of video tape take up a great deal of space and take a very long time to review. If the intention is to record procedures for teaching or for presentation at conference, then it is wise to set up a system for archiving the best examples and reusing tapes that contain nothing of interest. As a 1-h or 3-h tape may have one 10-min 'gem' recorded among the less good, it is necessary to have an 'edit suite' and a disciplined approach to archiving if the department is not to be swamped in video tape of mixed appeal. Whether the edit suite is shared with others or not, it is important to understand the basics of what it

can do and preferably for one of the medical team to learn how to use it in its most basic mode for compiling 'clips' of the best material or to make master tapes for the library and future use. The edit suite operates by recording from the original to a new tape in a sophisticated way. It must be able to play the same type of tape that has been chosen to record on in theatre, but it does not really matter if the edited master is of the same type or not (often the source machines are of more than one type and the mastering machine is of a high-quality format), as a copy of this on to tape of the original format can always be made. Edited masters should always be kept with the edit suite and seldom played, because they represent a great deal of work and the images are usually unrepeatable.

If access to an edit suite is routinely available, then a good system for collecting teaching material is to have a set of tapes in theatre and to record all the required procedures in a week. At the end of each week a member of the medical staff should take these tapes to the edit suite, compile on to a master tape all the excerpts that have been chosen and then mark the original tapes for re-use the following week. Most modern video cassettes can be re-used up to five times with absolutely no deterioration and such use can be indicated on the cassette label. In this way a good-quality and useful set of condensed master tapes will soon be created and a cassette (or two) for each day of the week is all that is ever in theatre. When a 'clip' is needed for a seminar or meeting, then this is quickly located and copied to the type of tape that is required. If a programme or presentation is to be made, then the edit suite can carry out sophisticated vision and sound editing. It is not likely that many medical staff will devote the time to being trained in the level of editing required for making programmes. This skill may be available in-house; if not, then a professional programme-maker should be consulted.

The editing and archiving of electronic still images is a craft that is yet to emerge, as much of the equipment is only just now becoming available. At present there are two types of machine for recording a video still: one is on a very small magnetic floppy disc which holds 50 images and can be rerecorded; the other is on a large laser disc which holds 72 000 images and can be recorded only once. The former has the advantage of low price and small discs (which could be kept with notes); the latter has the advantages of being computer compatible (it could be part of a patient record database) and is a permanent record. It is likely that one of two strategies for using such equipment will evolve: either the still images recorded from the endoscopic camera will be loaded to an inexpensive floppy disc in theatre and then taken to a central archive where selected images can be loaded to the optical disc and logged on the computer, or a link will be installed from the theatre to a central database, selected still images being recorded by way of this line direct to the optical disc, all under computer control that logs these images to the correct patient's file. With either of these two methods it is also possible to have a high-quality printer as part of the central facility to make either slides or prints at any time in the future from the recorded stills.

This will generally enhance the base of teaching images available with a relational database to enable them to be located quickly, previewed on a monitor and reproduced at the time, if required.

Physics of endoscopic technology

M. J. Coptcoat ChM, FRCS
Consultant Urologist, King's College Hospital, London, UK

Diathermy

Monopolar diathermy operates by producing an alternating current with wavelengths in the radio frequency range. The current passes through the patient's tissues from the active electrode, which is always small and in the form of a needle, blade, or forceps, to the indifferent electrode, which is usually a metal foil plate. There is a thermal effect beneath each electrode, but this is minimal beneath the large surface area of the indifferent electrode. The concentration of heat beneath the small active electrode is sufficient to coagulate the tissues. If the intensity of the current is increased, charring of the tissue (fulguration) will occur. A further increase of intensity will produce an arc between the tissues and the active electrode, leading to a cutting effect. The quality of the coagulation or cutting has been improved by the ability of newer machines to alter not only the frequency of oscillation but also the wave form. A smooth sine wave produces perfect cutting, while an interrupted burst provides excellent coagulation. A blended current is simply one that is half-way between these two extremes.

The indifferent electrode is now either a foil sheet or a self-adhesive plate with or without conductive jelly. It must be in uniform contact with the skin and should be sited such that the diathermy current does not traverse any of the cardiac electrical axes. The front of the thigh or under the buttock are probably the best sites for most urological procedures; they must be kept dry.

The active electrode is designed to meet the needs of the surgery being performed and usually takes the form of a point, blade, or loop. Coagulation and fulguration are better achieved with a slightly larger surface area in the form of a button or roller ball. Blood vessels are more efficiently sealed if diathermy is combined with coaptation, that is, holding the vessel wall together.

Modern pacemakers show much less response than older models, but as a precaution the indifferent electrode plate should be situated as far as possible from the pacemaker.

Diathermy in open surgery

1a, b Where diatherapy is used in any organ that has an end-artery type of blood supply, there may be a channelling effect of the current through that pedicle. This is particularly relevant when operating on the testicle and penis of a child. Monopolar diathermy can be used in these situations, but the organ must be placed directly in contact with the patient's thigh, so that the current can be conducted through this much larger contact area.

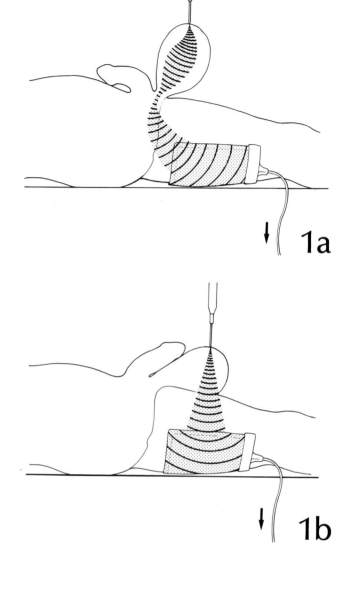

Diathermy in endoscopic surgery

Cutting and coagulation under fluid require higher currents. Normal saline may prevent the creation of a cutting arc because of its conductivity. Sterile water can be used, but is too readily absorbed by the body. Mannitol, urea, dextrose and glycine are suitable, safe irrigants. Unwanted adductor spasm during bladder resections can be lessened by either the infiltration of local anaesthetic or the use of a strong coagulant current in that area until the spasm ceases (neural exhaustion).

Capacitor suppression will be required on some diathermy units to allow the unimpaired use of endoscopic CCD cameras.

Bipolar diathermy

This is very useful in paediatric surgery. Bipolar forceps have each arm insulated and the current passes between the tips. It is therefore the safest form of diathermy, but at the present time a successful design has not been achieved for its application in endoscopic surgery.

Complications of diathermy

Diathermy can only be used at a legal minimum limit of 25 cm away from anaesthetic apparatus. The greatest risk of explosion occurs with the use of cyclopropane and ethers. This is even possible with modern venting systems. A more recently described complication is delayed explosion of gases within the urinary tract after diathermy. It is thought that this occurs because of inadvertent introduction of oxygen through the irrigation fluid in the form of bubbles. There have been case reports of explosions in both the bladder and kidney after fulguration of tumours which have led to extravasation. Every attempt should be made to avoid the introduction of air bubbles in irrigation fluid to minimize this risk.

High voltage electrocution of a patient is a very rare but lethal event and can only arise with faults within the diathermy machine. Many machines have buzzer alarms, and these must be strictly used and the machine immediately turned off and checked when the alarm is sounded.

Ignition of flammable material on the patient's skin usually occurs when ethanol preparations are used for skin sterilization. There is also the potential danger that even less flammable preparations may react with the aluminium diathermy earthing plate, producing intense chemical heat locally, and so the plate must always be kept free of such fluids.

Thermoelectric burns result from misuse of diathermy by the surgeon. The use of diathermy through other metal instruments, such as forceps, in open surgery must be very carefully observed to avoid wound contact. Irrigation fluid generally vastly decreases the thermal conduction of diathermy when used endoscopically, but it is still possible to cause damage to surrounding small intestine when fulgurating the bladder dome. Some patients are temporarily incontinent following transurethral resection of the prostate (TURP). This is probably due to excessive use of diathermy and a transient thermal injury to the sphincter mechanism. It is possible, though not proved, that some cases of impotence associated with TURP may also be due to thermal injury to the adjacent neurovascular bundle, but this can only be presumed in the absence of any psychological cause.

Lasers

The word LASER is an acronym for Light Amplification by Stimulated Emission of Radiation.

A laser is capable of generating an intense parallel beam of electromagnetic energy of a given wavelength or colour. Lasers are capable of generating light either in the form of a continuous delivery of energy, referred to as continuous-wave lasers, or in the form of discrete or multiple pulses, referred to as pulsed lasers. Laser wavelengths cover the entire visible portion of the electromagnetic spectrum, as well as wavelengths in the ultraviolet and infrared portions. Lasers differ primarily in the wavelength of the light emitted by the active medium. The absorption coefficient of tissues varies according to the wavelength; thus, the thermal changes in the tissue and penetration depth of the incident beam depend on the wavelength of light chosen.

The application of lasers for endoscopic surgery is dependent on the ability to transmit laser energy through the instrument. This is facilitated by the use of the fine quartz fibres in the majority of cases. *Table 1* lists the lasers most commonly used in urology and their characteristics.

Indications for lasers

Lesions of the external genitalia

Condylomata that are refractory to treatment with topical agents can be treated with the carbon dioxide, neodymium yttrium aluminium garnet (NdYAG), or argon laser with equal success. The NdYAG laser appears to be the superior laser for treating penile carcinoma, because it possesses a greater depth of penetration with less tissue disruption. Haemangiomata are best treated with the argon laser, because its emission is preferentially absorbed by haemoglobin.

Table 1 Characteristics of lasers in common urological use

Laser	Wavelength (nm)	Mode	Delivery system	Comment
Carbon dioxide	10 600	Continuous-wave and pulsed	Wave-guide	Minimal absorption. Good for cutting
NdYAG*	1064	Continuous-wave and pulsed	Fibreoptic	Minimal absorption (5–6 mm). Good for tissue destruction and small vessel haemostasis
Argon	458–515	Continuous-wave and pulsed	Fibreoptic	Absorbed by haemoglobin
Dye	400–700	Continuous-wave and pulsed	Fibreoptic	Variable wavelength. Lithotripsy in pulsed mode

*Neodymium yttrium aluminium garnet

Vasovasostomy

With the addition of a milliwatt adaptor, the carbon dioxide laser can be used as a tissue welder. Two or three stay sutures are still required, but it is a quicker technique than a microsurgical anastomosis and the overall results are similar.

Superficial bladder tumours

The NdYAG laser has the potential to be used with either a rigid or a flexible cystoscope. Theoretical advantages and animal experiments suggest that the laser should be safer and more accurate than traditional electrocautery, but this has not been borne out by the majority of clinical series. The best place for the laser remains as an adjunct to outpatient flexible cystoscopy with local anaesthesia.

Superficial tumours of the upper urinary tract

The fine flexible quartz fibre of the delivery system makes it an ideal tool to be used through a flexible ureteroscope or nephroscope for superficial transitional cell carcinomas. A separate biopsy will also be required.

Photodynamic therapy for bladder cancer

This involves the intravenous administration of an agent that is selectively taken up by the tumour tissue, so making the tissue more susceptible to detection and to injury when illuminated by certain wavelengths of light. The most commonly used sensitizing agent is a haematoporphyrin derivative. Cytotoxicity occurs in cells that have taken up the haematoporphyrin derivative when they are exposed to wavelengths of lights corresponding to the peaks on the absorption spectrum of the derivative. A gold metal vapour laser or the argon laser are the types commonly used for this type of treatment. Unfortunately, patients experience a marked skin photosensitivity during treatment, and until more specific sensitizers are available, photodynamic therapy will not gain widespread acceptance.

Lithotripsy

Extracorporeal shock wave lithotripsy is the first-choice treatment for the majority of intrarenal and ureteric calculi. There are many instances, however, when an impacted stone is recalcitrant to such treatment or a lithotripter may not be available. In these cases, the treatment of choice is ureteroscopy and laser lithotripsy. The pulsed dye laser uses a wavelength preferentially absorbed by the stone. A plasma is formed on the stone surface, resulting in a photoacoustic coupling phenomenon that fragments the stone. This can only occur with pulsed laser light. This is far superior to both electrohydraulic and ultrasonographic lithotripsy in the confined space of the ureter.

Electrohydraulic disintegration

An electrohydraulic phenomenon can be created at the tip of a small probe and used to fragment a urinary stone through the working channel of either a ureteroscope or a nephroscope. The electrohydraulic probe produces a shock wave, which is created by an underwater explosion from an ultrashort electrical discharge between two closely approximated electrodes. If two electrodes are placed in a fluid medium and a high tension voltage discharged between them for a very short time, the fluid will be vaporized and a bubble will be generated that will spread out at the speed of sound. If a stone is close to this site of discharge, the outer surface of the stone will create a change in the impedance of the wave. This will produce tension and compression waves through the stone, resulting in its fragmentation if the coefficient of material strength can be overcome.

2 The electrodes are manufactured in two types: coaxial and parallel.

Such probes provide a very efficient method for localized endoscopic stone fragmentation. The larger the probe, the greater is the potential shock wave; probes of 9-Fr gauge are used through a nephroscope, and probes of 5-Fr, 3-Fr and 2-Fr gauge are available for ureteroscopic use.

Any proximity of the probe tip to the urothelium may lead to perforation, and so great accuracy of placement must be achieved. This demands excellent visualization of the probe tip, stone and surrounding urothelium, which is easy to obtain in the intrarenal collecting system or bladder, but difficult in the ureter.

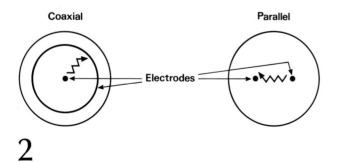

Coaxial   Parallel

Electrodes

2

Ultrasonic disintegration

This method for endoscopic stone fragmentation differs from electrohydraulic and laser lithotripsy in that the mechanism is one of drilling. Ultrasonic drilling of calculi involves the piezoelectric excitation of a quartz crystal to make it expand and contract and thus produce a vibration energy. Increasing the frequency of an applied alternating potential causes the crystal to vibrate at high speed with production of a sine wave displacement.

3 Transmission of this vibration to a metal probe or cylinder will cause the probe to vibrate in sympathy. Probe tip movement will be maximal if the maximum amplitude of the sine wave is coincident with the tip of the probe. Worn probes are therefore less efficient.

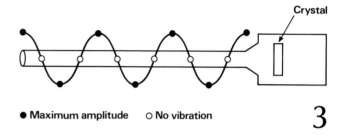

● Maximum amplitude   ○ No vibration

3

Small fragments are broken from a stone as the tip is applied. The probe must be used through a rigid instrument and so there must be an offset eyepiece for that endoscope.

If the working probe is hollow, the fragments can be sucked away. This provides a great advantage over all other forms of extracorporeal and intracorporeal lithotripsy, which rely on the spontaneous passage of a fragmented stone. The probes are available as 9-Fr gauge for nephroscopic application and as 5-Fr gauge for the ureteroscope. A 1-Fr gauge solid probe is available for some miniature ureteroscopes.

A considerable amount of energy is converted to heat if the probe is used in long bursts. This requires an efficient flow of irrigation fluid around the probe during its use. Ultrasonic lithotripsy is not suitable for very hard stones, such as cystine and calcium oxalate mono-hydrate. In these cases it can be used in combination with electrohydraulic lithotripsy, where an initial bore hole is made with the ultrasonic probe, which will then allow the effective placement of the electrohydraulic probe within that hole, rather like the method employed for dynamite.

Further reading

McNicholas TA, ed. *Lasers in Urology. Principles and Practice.* London: Springer-Verlag, 1990.

Miller RA. Endoscopic application of shock wave technology for the destruction of renal calculi. *World J Urol* 1985; 3: 36–40.

Mitchell JP, Lumb GN, Dobbie AK. *A Handbook of Surgical Diathermy.* 2nd edn. Bristol: John Wright, 1978.

Fundamentals of shock wave production in lithotripsy

A. J. Coleman MSc, PhD
Principal Physicist, Medical Physics Department, St Thomas' Hospital, London, UK

History

Early attempts to disintegrate human calculi with acoustic energy were reported by Lamport *et al.* in 1950[1]. They used continuous wave ultrasound from a piezoelectric source directed from a distance at a stone suspended in water. With this arrangement, however, the exposure required for complete stone fragmentation generates unacceptable heating of any intervening tissue. The clinical use of continuous wave ultrasound in lithotripsy was therefore confined to treatments in which the acoustic source could be placed in close contact with the stone.

1 High amplitude acoustic pulses, known as shock waves, were also identified in the early 1950s as being capable of fragmenting brittle objects. Such pulses were generated electrohydraulically by inducing an electrical discharge between a pair of submerged electrodes and were used by Goldberg in 1959 for close contact fragmentation of bladder stones[2]. Hausler and Kiefer[3] in 1971 were the first to demonstrate the potential use of shock waves in contact-free lithotripsy and it was soon realized that the use of pulses could reduce the problem of tissue heating, which was found to result from continuous wave, contact-free exposure.

Shock wave sources suitable for the initial biological and ultimate clinical studies on contact-free shock wave lithotripsy were developed by the Dornier Company of West Germany. A Dornier prototype electrohydraulic shock wave source was employed by Chaussy for the early animal studies on contact-free lithotripsy at the Institute for Surgical Research, University of Munich,

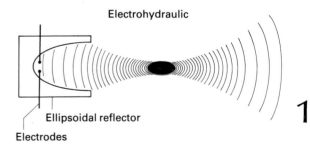

Electrohydraulic

Ellipsoidal reflector

Electrodes

1

throughout the 1970s[4]. These studies laid the foundation for the clinical treatment that is now known as extracorporeal shock wave lithotripsy (ESWL) and the first human patient was treated by Chaussy in 1980 at the University of Munich's Department of Urology using the Dornier Human Model 1 (HM-1) lithotripter.

Principles

Shock waves

2 The acoustic pulses employed in ESWL are distorted from the familiar representation of sound as a sinusoidally varying pressure disturbance with a single frequency and velocity. The distortion occurs because, at sufficiently high pressures, the peak of the wave propagates faster than the trough. As a result, the leading edge of the wave tends to develop an almost discontinuous step as it advances. Such a pulse is known as a shock wave and can be described in terms of a range of frequencies with a fundamental frequency (typically 150 kHz in ESWL) and a number of higher harmonics. The shock wave is more usually described in the literature on ESWL in terms of parameters such as the peak values of the acoustic pressure, the rise time of the shock front and the width of the pulse.

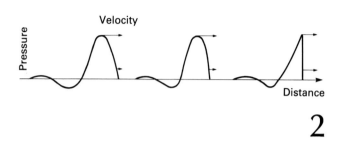

2

Shock wave generation

The generation of a spherically expanding waterborne shock wave requires the rapid release of sufficient energy within a small volume of water and may be achieved by the detonation of a small explosive pellet or the induction of an electrical spark between a closely spaced pair of electrodes. These violent processes are typically accompanied by an audible 'crack'. A water

vapour bubble expands and pushes the water ahead of it. As the resulting shock wave spreads out, its peak pressure decreases, and in order to obtain the pressures needed to fragment a stone the wave must be focused. This is done for point sources by reflecting the expanding wave at an ellipsoidal surface.

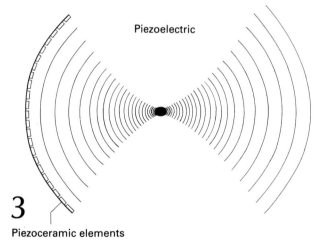

Piezoelectric

3

Piezoceramic elements

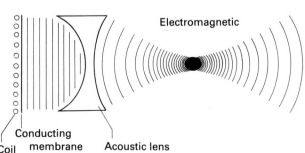

Electromagnetic

Coil Conducting membrane Acoustic lens

4

3,4 Extended, as opposed to point, sources of acoustic energy are available in the form of piezoelectric and electromagnetic acoustic transducers, and are also employed to generate shock waves. High pressures are obtained by driving these transducers with a large amplitude, electrical impulse and focusing the resulting acoustic pulse. A piezoelectric source may consist of a spherical array of piezoceramic elements which, when driven, emit an acoustic pulse that converges at the centre of curvature of the array. An electromagnetic source may take the form of a plane disc of metal foil which flexes rapidly when an electrical pulse is applied to an adjacent flat coil. The plane wave from this source is then focused by an acoustic lens. The pulse from extended sources, in contrast to point sources, typically becomes shocked only as the pulse nears the focus.

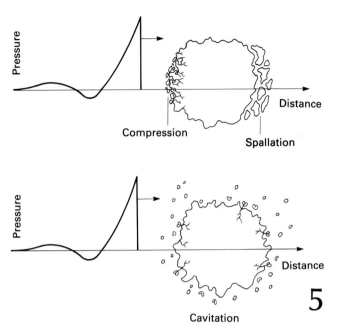

Stone fragmentation

5 Two effects known as spallation and cavitation are most commonly cited as the mechanisms of shock wave fragmentation of stones in ESWL. Spallation occurs when a wave travelling in a brittle material such as stone is internally reflected. On reflection the wave acquires an enhanced tensile component and the stone, which is weaker in tension than in compression, tends to fragment close to this reflecting surface.

Cavitation involves the nucleation, enlargement and collapse of bubbles in a fluid and may be induced by the shock wave in fluid surrounding the stone. This effect occurs only when the tensile component of the shock wave is greater then the tensile strength of the fluid. The collapse of the cavities within the fluid is a violent process which generates further shock waves and high speed liquid jets which are both capable of eroding the stone.

Operation of lithotripters

The principal skill required of the lithotripter operator is in the use of the imaging system to visualize the stone, locate it at the position of the shock wave focus, and assess when fragmentation is complete. This presupposes good quality radiographic or ultrasonographic images and precise alignment of the imaging system with the shock wave focus. Along with an ability to interpret these images, the operator must rely on experience to select the output setting of the shock wave generator and the maximum number of shock wave pulses appropriate for a given case. In the absence of a universally accepted physical definition of acoustic exposure in ESWL, the appropriate output setting and number of shocks required on each particular lithotripter can be judged only by experience.

References

1. Lamport H, Newman HF, Eichhorn RD. Fragmentation of biliary calculi by ultrasound. *Fed Proc* 1950; 9: 73–4.

2. Goldberg V. Eine neue methode der harnsteinzertrunerung – elektrohydralische lithotripsie. *Urologe B* 1959; 19: 23–7.

3. Hausler E, Kiefer W. Anregung von stobwellen in flussigkeiten durch hochgeschwindigkeitswassertriopfen. *Verb Dtsch Physikal Ges* 1971; 6: 786.

4. Chaussy C. (ed.) *Extracorporeal Shock Wave Lithotripsy*. Basel: Karger, 1982.

Illustrations by Paul Richardson

Needle nephrostomy

I. B. Nockler FRCR
Consultant Radiologist, St Bartholomew's Hospital, London, UK

History

The percutaneous puncture of kidneys was first carried out in 1934, but the technique developed very slowly over the next four decades. The technique of percutaneous nephrostomy as we now practise it was introduced in the mid 1970s[1] and was initially considered as a substitute for surgical decompression in very ill patients before definitive surgery. Further development and expansion occurred as the result of technical advances in catheter and guidewire materials as well as the impact of modern imaging modalities.

Principles and justification

Indications

Obstruction

Simple obstruction of a kidney may be tolerated for about a week but the likelihood of reversible renal failure decreases as the duration of obstruction progresses. Where obstruction is unlikely to reverse spontaneously or in an infected kidney or in renal failure, immediate drainage should be established. The causes of obstruction are usually a stone or malignancy of pelvic or urothelial origin.

Diversion

Urinary diversion by percutaneous nephrostomy in strictures or leaks is an effective and simple way of allowing healing of postoperative wounds or ureteric fistulae. This may be of particular value in transplanted kidneys with early or late complications of obstruction or leaks.

Access for further interventional procedures

The placing of a percutaneous nephrostomy tube allows a safe and convenient route to the renal collecting system for endourological procedures including stent placement and stone removal.

Contraindications

There are no absolute contraindications to the procedure. Uncorrected coagulopathy is a relative contraindication, but in a urosepticaemic patient with disseminated intravascular coagulopathy drainage is mandatory.

Preoperative

Good radiological evaluation is essential and is likely to be the basis for determining the status of the renal collecting system. A recent urogram and ultrasonographic examination must be available and computed tomography may be required to assess optimal placement of a nephrostomy tube, to avoid causing visceral damage. This may be particularly important in horseshoe kidneys and in severe kyphoscoliosis and splenomegaly.

Informed consent must be obtained and the haemoglobin and clotting screen performed if stone extraction is planned. Antibiotics are given if urinary infection exists and if calculi are present.

Premedication is not usually needed unless nephrostomy precedes stone removal under general anaesthesia. Small amounts of diazepam and pethidine hydrochloride may be given but severely uraemic patients may not need sedation.

Operations

Position of patient

1 Patient positioning is important. Normally access is provided with the patient in the prone or prone oblique position. The latter is favoured as it provides easy access to the collecting system if only fluoroscopic guidance is utilized. The position may need to be modified in patients with severe kyphoscoliosis.

Renal transplant patients are placed in the supine position to allow access to the superficially placed kidney in the anterolateral abdomen.

Image guidance

The positioning of the nephrostomy tube under fluoroscopic guidance is the most widely used method and is necessary for accurate guidewire and catheter manipulations.

Ultrasonographic guidance for the initial puncture is useful in dilated collecting systems, where the system fails to opacify after intravenous contrast, in pregnancy (when irradiation is undesirable) and in patients with a history of contrast medium reactions. Ultrasonography alone may be used but only in dilated systems.

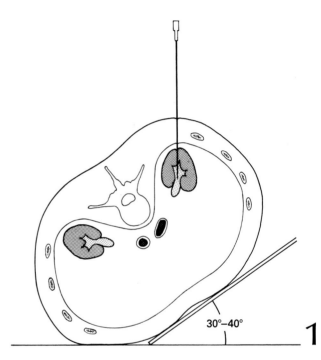

30°–40°

1

ANGIOGRAPHIC (SELDINGER) TECHNIQUE

The Seldinger technique involves puncturing the collecting system, inserting a guidewire through the sheath, dilating the tract and exchanging the dilator for the drainage catheter over the guidewire.

The author favours an initial puncture of the collecting system with a 22-Fr Chiba needle to perform an antegrade study if the collecting system is not already opacified and to assess the depth and angle of optimal puncture for drainage. This is performed after infiltrating the tract with about 10 ml of local anaesthetic.

2 For drainage of the system, a lower pole calix is preferred for puncture, and when possible the tract should be inferior to the 12th rib. If stone removal or stent placement is to follow, a middle or upper calix may need to be punctured, increasing the risk of a pneumothorax.

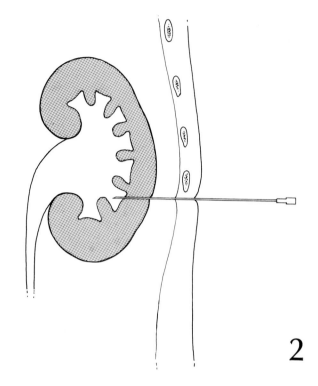

2

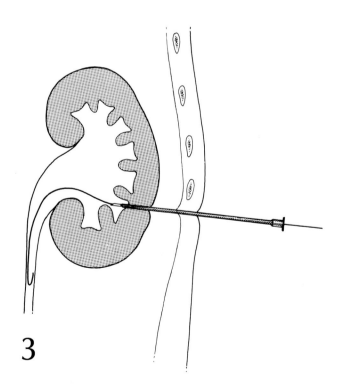

3

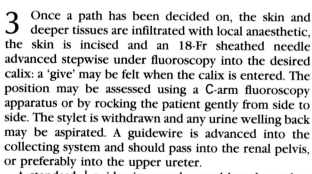

3 Once a path has been decided on, the skin and deeper tissues are infiltrated with local anaesthetic, the skin is incised and an 18-Fr sheathed needle advanced stepwise under fluoroscopy into the desired calix: a 'give' may be felt when the calix is entered. The position may be assessed using a C-arm fluoroscopy apparatus or by rocking the patient gently from side to side. The stylet is withdrawn and any urine welling back may be aspirated. A guidewire is advanced into the collecting system and should pass into the renal pelvis, or preferably into the upper ureter.

A standard J guidewire may be used but the author favours a stiffer Lunderquist exchange wire. Occasionally a Bentson wire is utilized if the infundibulum to a calix is narrow, the floppy end facilitating entry into the pelvis.

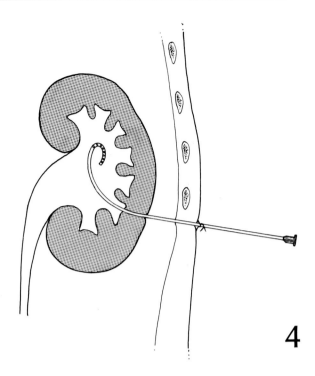

4   The sheath is withdrawn and the tract dilated over the guidewire to 8 Fr to the site of entry into the collecting system. A 7-Fr pigtail nephrostomy catheter is advanced into the renal pelvis over the guidewire. Once the drainage catheter is satisfactorily placed, the guidewire is removed. An antegrade study may be performed at this stage, but if the urine is infected this should be delayed until the infection has cleared.

4

TROCAR–CANNULA/CATHETER TECHNIQUE

Patient positioning, opacification of the collecting system, selection of entry tract and imaging guidance are the same as for the Seldinger technique. A small skin incision is made and a 10-Fr trocar–cannula advanced under fluoroscopic control into the desired calix. Urine drains from the trocar when it lies within the collecting system. The trocar is removed and a soft 8-Fr catheter passed through the cannula into the renal pelvis.

NEEDLE CATHETER METHOD

This technique involves a catheter placed over a needle trocar which is then introduced into the collecting system. The catheter is advanced over the needle trocar and the trocar is withdrawn, leaving the catheter within the renal pelvis. Cope loop catheters and Sack's Elecath fluid-draining systems are useful in dilated systems where dislodgement may be a problem.

Once the drainage catheter of choice is in position, firm fixation with silk or nylon sutures to the skin is important.

Postoperative care

All patients are hospitalized overnight and checked for bleeding and sepsis and urine output. Initial observations are every 30 min for 2 h, then hourly for 2 h, followed by 4-hourly observations.

Complications

Bleeding

Transient haematuria may be expected. Occasionally clots may form in the collecting system, potentially obstructing the nephrostomy tube; saline irrigation should clear the system. If bleeding is severe and a fall in packed cell volume occurs, ultrasonographic examination should be performed to exclude retroperitoneal bleeding. Gross haematuria may indicate arterial damage.

Infection

Septicaemia may develop, especially if the nephrostomy was carried out for pyonephrosis. Perinephric abscesses are rare.

Urinoma

This may occasionally be encountered but rarely requires any specific treatment.

Pneumothorax

This should not occur if inferior pole calices are punctured, but can occur with more cranial puncture sites.

Catheter-related problems

Dislodgement
The dressings should not be disturbed and no traction applied to the catheter. If the catheter is accidentally dislodged drainage should be reinstituted as soon as possible, especially if infection is present. An attempt should be made to use the previous tract but a new puncture site may have to be made.

Obstruction of the catheter
In the presence of clear urine catheter irrigation may not be necessary, but when blood clot, pus or debris obstructs the catheter, gentle irrigation with saline should be attempted. Inserting a guidewire will clear more stubborn obstructions, but occasionally it may be necessary to insert a new catheter over a guidewire.

Outcome

In trained hands percutaneous nephrostomy is successful in 98% of patients. The complication rate is less than 4%, most being minor. Short-term renal failure due to obstruction may be reversed to near-normal function.

Long-standing failure is less predictable and drainage may need to be extended to assess final renal function.

Drainage for decompression yields good results and a number of endourological procedures can follow safe and reliable percutaneous access.

Reference

1. Pfister RC, Newhouse JH. Interventional percutaneous pyelo-ureteral techniques. II. Percutaneous nephrostomy and other procedures. *Radiol Clin North Am* 1979; 17: 351–63.

Further reading

Barbaric ZL, Davis RS, Frank IN, Linke CA, Lipchik EO, Cockett ATK. Percutaneous nephropyelostomy in the management of acute pyohydronephrosis. *Radiology* 1976; 118: 567–73.

Fowler JE, Meares EM Jr, Goldin AR. Percutaneous nephrostomy: techniques, indications and results. *Urology* 1975; 6: 428–34.

Goodwin WE, Casey WC, Woolf W. Percutaneous trocar (needle) nephrostomy in hydronephrosis. *JAMA* 1955; 157: 891–4.

Pedersen JF, Cowan DF, Kristensen JK *et al.* Ultrasonically guided percutaneous nephrostomy: report of 24 cases. *Radiology* 1976; 119: 429–31.

Reznek RH, Talner LB. Percutaneous nephrostomy. *Radiol Clin North Am* 1984; 22: 393–406.

Illustrations by Paul Richardson

Percutaneous nephrolithotomy

H. N. Whitfield MA, MChir, FRCS
Consultant Urologist, St Bartholomew's Hospital and St Mark's Hospital for Diseases of the Colon and Rectum, London, UK

History

The first occasion on which a renal stone was extracted percutaneously as a planned procedure through a track formed for the purpose was in 1976[1]. The track had been dilated slowly over a number of days, but it quickly became apparent that a track could safely be dilated to 30-Fr gauge in one stage and the stone removed at the same sitting. With the advent of extracorporeal shock wave lithotripsy (ESWL) percutaneous nephrolithotomy has become incorporated as part of the combined management of complex stones, and also as a technique to overcome complications of lithotripsy.

Principles and justification

Indications

Almost any stone, irrespective of its size, composition and situation, can be removed by a percutaneous technique. Large, complex stones may require two or more tracks and the procedure can become very prolonged, in which case open surgery may be a viable alternative, particularly if there has been no previous surgery. If ESWL is available, the policy of debulking a large stone percutaneously and then treating the rest by ESWL is well established.

Contraindications

Although there are no absolute contraindications to a percutaneous nephrolithotomy there are some occasions on which the procedure is associated with difficulties. Access in patients with a severe kyphoscoliosis may be complicated, even on occasions requiring a planned transpleural approach. Ultrasonography and computed tomographic scanning may facilitate initial access to the collecting system in patients with horse-shoe kidneys and in those with a severe kyphoscoliosis. Such patients will, however, pose similar problems for both open surgery and ESWL. Very hard stones, such as uric acid or cystine stones, can be difficult and slow to disintegrate, and access to stones in upper pole calices can be difficult.

Preoperative

The result of a recent urine culture and a full blood count must be available. Overall renal function should be measured by serum creatinine, and if there is diminished function the precise level should be established by measurement of creatinine clearance, and the differential renal function ascertained by isotope renography. An intravenous urogram is needed to demonstrate pelvicaliceal anatomy and a plain radiograph on the day of surgery is essential.

Parenteral antibiotics should be given to all patients prophylactically and if the stone is infective in origin a more prolonged course of an oral antibiotic, for up to 3 months, is indicated.

Operation

The patient should be intubated and ventilated and intravenous fluid is required for at least 24 h after the operation.

The formation of the track is performed initially as for a needle nephrostomy, save that a retrograde ureteric catheter is first passed, through which contrast can be injected to opacify and to fill the pelvicaliceal system. The presence of the ureteric catheter helps to prevent stone fragments from falling into the ureter, and allows ready identification of the pelviureteric junction.

1a, b The track is dilated up to approximately 30-Fr gauge with either a series of graded polytetrafluoroethylene dilators or with a telescopic metal bougie system. This latter has the advantage that the track remains continuously tamponaded, thereby reducing or eliminating bleeding into the collecting system; the disadvantage is that the dilators are snub-nosed and difficult to insert in a muscular patient or after previous surgery. The size of the track is determined by the size of the instrument that will be used. It is seldom necessary for the track to be larger than 30 Fr; the size of most instruments necessitates a minimum of 26 Fr. An Amplatz sheath is inserted over the dilator to maintain a track of the chosen size.

Normal saline warmed to body temperature is the irrigant, which should be used to reduce the possibility of 'TUR (transurethral resection) syndrome' if extravasation occurs.

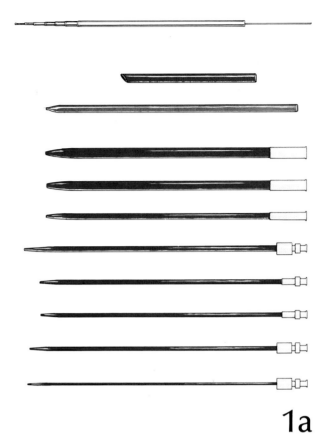

1a

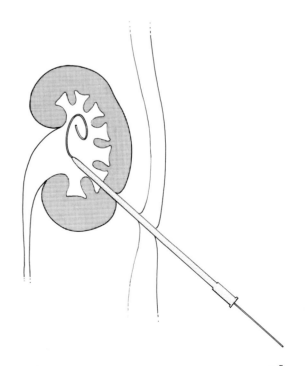

1b

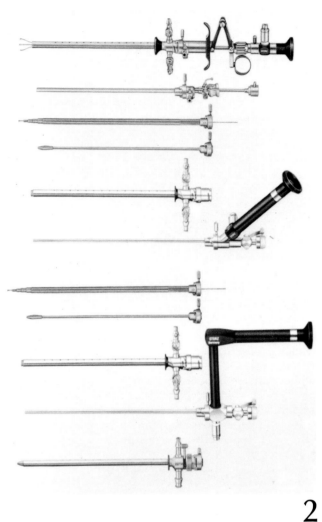

2 A variety of nephroscopes is available, most of which have an offset eyepiece to enable operating instruments to utilize a straight channel.

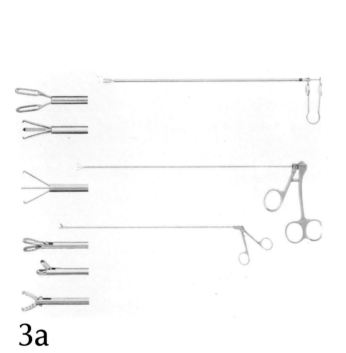

3a

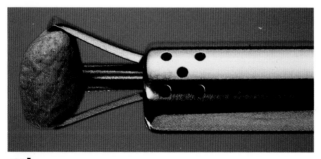

3b

3a, b Stones which are small enough to be removed intact can be grasped with a stone forceps. Larger stones need to be disintegrated electrohydraulically or with ultrasound (*see* pp. 27–31).

4a–d Stones in the renal pelvis are readily accessible; some stones in upper pole calices can be reached, but stones in middle calices may be difficult to visualize.

If there is difficulty visualizing a stone, fluoroscopy can be employed to relate the stone to the tip of the instrument. At the end of the procedure, stone clearance should be confirmed both visually and radiographically.

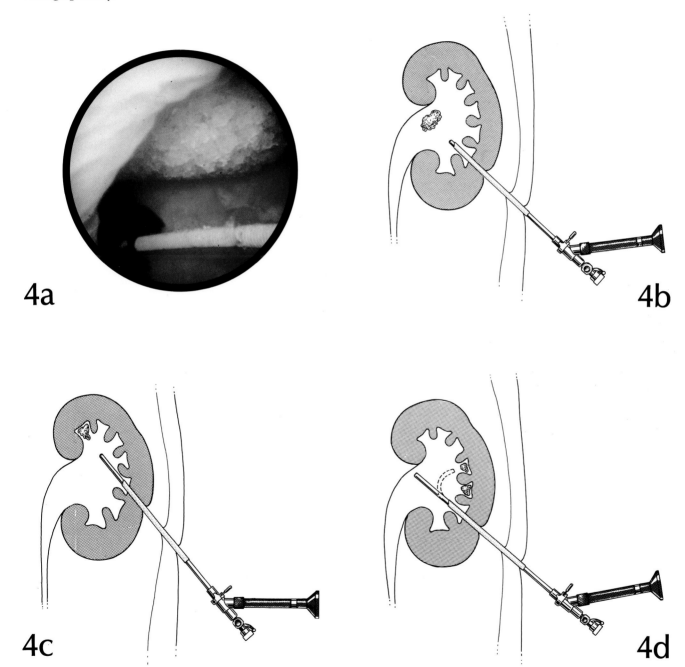

4a

4b

4c

4d

Postoperative care

5   At the end of the procedure a nephrostomy tube of the same size as the Amplatz sheath should be left in place for 24–48 h to tamponade the track. When the urine is clear the nephrostomy tube should be clamped. A nephrostogram is not essential if the procedure was uncomplicated, and a postoperative radiograph confirms the absence of all stones. If loin pain, fever or leakage around the nephrostomy tube occurs, urinary drainage should be replaced and a nephrostogram performed.

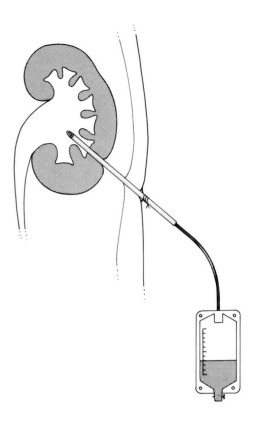

5

Complications

In spite of prophylactic antibiotics septicaemia may arise, especially when operating on stones which are infective in origin. Supportive measures must be employed vigorously, and parenteral antibiotic treatment with aminoglycosides or third generation cephalosporins instituted according to the sensitivities of any organisms which are isolated.

Extravasation of large volumes of irrigating fluid can occur if the collecting system is perforated. Intravascular leakage is more dangerous than perinephric extravasation. Intraperitoneal extravasation is also a possible hazard, and will provoke profound biochemical disturbance very rapidly. For these reasons the volume of irrigant being used and the volume retrieved must be monitored during the operation. If a discrepancy occurs the procedure should be brought to a halt, a nephrostomy tube inserted and completion postponed until a nephrostogram demonstrates no further leakage.

6a, b All precautions should be taken to ensure protection from irradiation. Screening times should be minimized, and irradiation reduced by using pulsed fluoroscopy, coned and stored images.

The exposure rate, especially to the head and neck of the operator, from under-couch screening apparatus is less than for over-couch equipment. Shielding is provided by the steel tabletop when the tube is below; the lead shielding is used to further reduce scattered X-rays from reaching operators. Lead shielding should be placed around the tube in over-couch tables to reduce scatter to the operator, as these tables are primarily meant for remote-control screening.

Fragments of stone which have passed down the ureter may need to be removed endoscopically. Retained fragments in the upper third of the ureter are best approached by antegrade ureteroscopy, but those in the lower two-thirds by retrograde ureteroscopy.

Bleeding can occur at the time of track dilatation, as a result of intrarenal manipulations or as secondary haemorrhage but such events are not common. Bleeding from the track is best controlled by the Amplatz sheath. At the end of the procedure a large-bore nephrostomy tube will serve the same purpose. If the bleeding is excessively heavy then the tube should be spigotted to provide additional tamponade. Anti-fibrinolytic agents should be avoided, since they result in very rubbery clots which are difficult to evacuate or to pass spontaneously. If bleeding becomes heavy enough to obscure vision, the procedure should be abandoned, with a view to being completed 72–96 h later.

Absorption of large quantities of irrigating fluid can occur. For this reason the volume of irrigant being used must be monitored constantly and titrated against the volume which is retrieved. Any gross discrepancy is an indication for abandoning the procedure. A 'TUR' reaction can arise, but should be avoided by using normal saline (at body temperature to prevent reduction of core temperature) and by following the guidelines above.

Residual stone fragments can be ignored if they are smaller than 3 mm in diameter. Fragments larger than this require either ESWL or a second-look procedure.

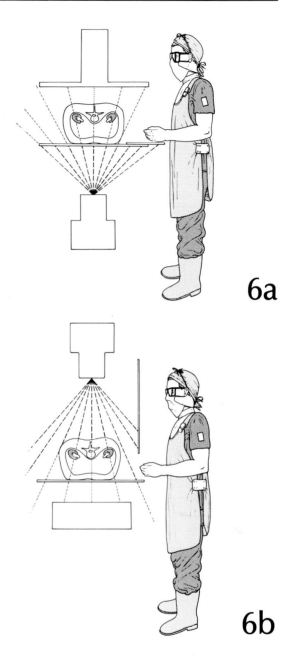

6a

6b

Outcome

The large majority of renal stones can be removed by this technique. Complex branched stones may necessitate more than one track; this is fully justifiable if ESWL is not available.

References

1. Fernström I, Johansson B. Percutaneous pyelolithotomy: a new extraction technique. *Scand J Urol Nephrol* 1976; 10: 257–9.

Further reading

Marberger M, Stackl W, Hruby W, Kroiss A. Late sequelae of ultrasonic lithotripsy of renal calculi. *J Urol* 1985; 133: 170–3.

Segura JW, Patterson DE, LeRoy AJ *et al.* Percutaneous removal of kidney stones: review of 1000 cases. *J Urol* 1985; 134: 1077–81.

Whitfield HN. Percutaneous nephrolithotomy. *Br J Urol* 1983; 55: 609–12.

Whitfield HN. Percutaneous stone removal techniques. In: Gingell C, Abrams P, eds. *Controversies and Innovations in Urological Surgery*. London: Springer, 1988: 35–45.

Wickham JEA, Miller RA, Kellet MJ. Percutaneous nephrolithotomy, results and cost effectiveness. *Br J Urol* 1983; Supplement: 103–6.

Pyelolysis/endopyelotomy

H. N. Whitfield MA, MChir, FRCS
Consultant Urologist, St Bartholomew's Hospital and St Mark's Hospital for Diseases of the Colon and Rectum, London, UK

History

The technique of percutaneous pyelolysis for pelvi-ureteric junction (PUJ) obstruction was first described in the UK in 1983 by Wickham[1,2], but was subsequently renamed endopyelotomy in North America. The principle depends on the regeneration of urothelium into a tube, which was demonstrated by Davis[3] to occur even in the presence of a full thickness defect in part of the circumference of the ureter.

Indications

PUJ obstruction, both primary idiopathic and secondary to infection, stones or previous surgery, may be treated by this method, although there is some difference in opinion about the relative merits of the procedure in the two broad categories of the condition. The technique is particularly useful in the presence of PUJ obstruction complicated by renal stones.

Preoperative

A high-dose frusemide intravenous urogram and an isotopic renogram should be performed before the operation to establish the diagnosis. A urine culture and an estimate of overall renal function are essential.

Operation

A retrograde wire must be passed across the PUJ into the renal pelvis. This can be difficult if the upper ureter is very tortuous, but a Bentson wire with a very soft, flexible tip can usually be guided into position. A 6-Fr angiocatheter is then passed over the guidewire into the renal pelvis. If this first step proves impossible, the procedure should be abandoned and an open operation performed.

1   To enable the PUJ region to be visualized easily and subsequently incised, a nephrostomy track is established and dilated to 28 Fr through a middle or upper calix, rather than a lower pole calix. An Amplatz sheath is passed over the dilator to maintain the track. The retrograde guidewire is pulled out from the renal pelvis along the Amplatz sheath with a pair of alligator forceps down a nephroscope.

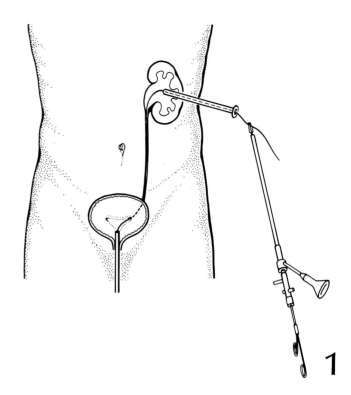

1

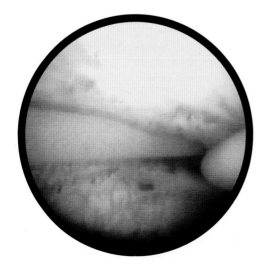

2

2   A second guidewire is inserted antegradely down the ureter alongside the retrograde angiocatheter.

3   A second angiocatheter is then passed over this guidewire to stretch the PUJ.

3

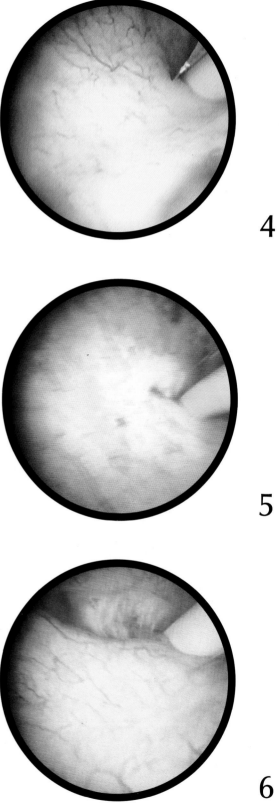

4

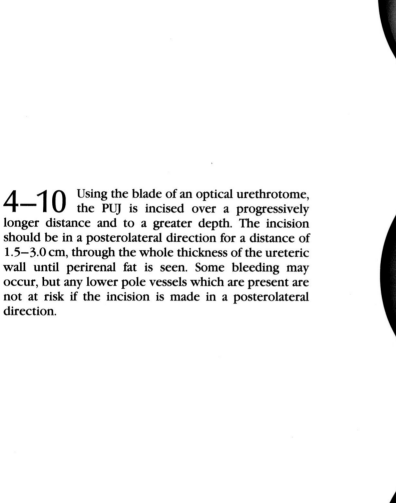

4–10 Using the blade of an optical urethrotome, the PUJ is incised over a progressively longer distance and to a greater depth. The incision should be in a posterolateral direction for a distance of 1.5–3.0 cm, through the whole thickness of the ureteric wall until perirenal fat is seen. Some bleeding may occur, but any lower pole vessels which are present are not at risk if the incision is made in a posterolateral direction.

5

6

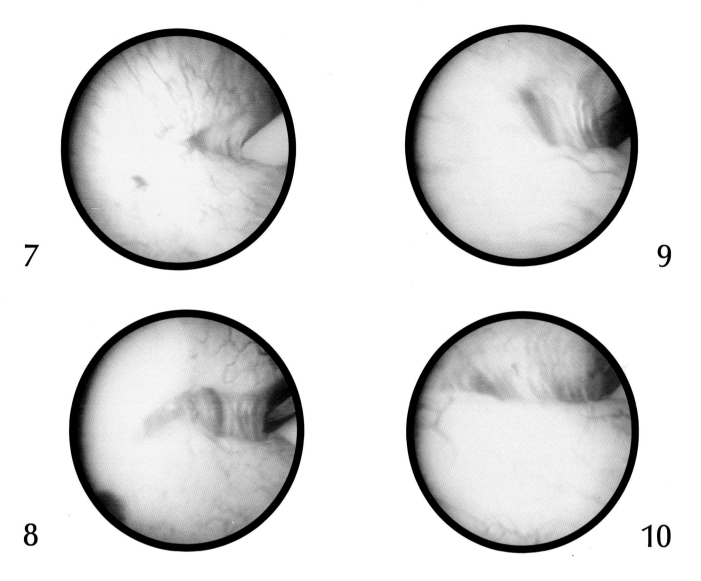

7

9

8

10

11 To hold the PUJ open during healing and to prevent healing across the junction from occurring from side to side, a 12–14-Fr diameter stent should be introduced over one of the guidewires. To avoid external drainage the most satisfactory form of stent for this purpose is a modified JJ stent which has an expanded upper end. This should be introduced over the guidewire which has been inserted antegradely to prevent the distal end of the stent from entering the urethra. However, the retrograde guidewire should be left *in situ* during the insertion of the JJ stent. If difficulty is encountered during stent insertion, it is helpful to use the retrograde guidewire which can be held taut proximally and distally. Great care must be taken to ensure that the distal end of the JJ stent remains in the bladder. The position of the distal end of the stent should be checked fluoroscopically, and that of the proximal end checked both fluoroscopically and visually.

If a modified JJ stent of the kind described is not available, two 6-Fr JJ stents may be inserted antegradely with equal effect using the two guidewires.

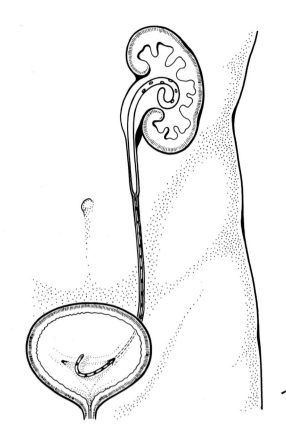

11

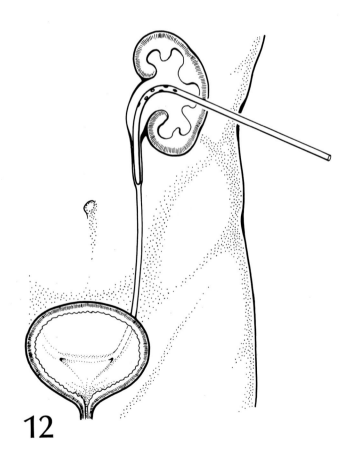

12

12 An alternative is to use a modified nephrostomy tube which passes across the PUJ and is brought out through the nephrostomy track. Side holes in the tube where it lies within the renal pelvis ensure that urinary drainage can occur either to an external collecting bag or, if the nephrostomy tube is spigotted, urine will pass down into the ureter.

Postoperative care

A 28-Fr nephrostomy tube should be left for 24–48 h to tamponade the track. A urethral catheter should remain for 72 h to prevent extravasation of urine at the pyelotomy during micturition when free reflux up the JJ stent will inevitably occur.

13 If the stent that has been inserted is of the variety shown in *Illustration 12*, a urethral catheter is unnecessary. A large size nephrostomy tube can be introduced over the stent from 48 h to tamponade the nephrostomy track. Care must be taken not to dislodge the stent when removing the nephrostomy tube. The stent should be grasped by a pair of alligator forceps and pushed inwards while the nephrostomy tube is pulled out over the alligator forceps. The stent can be spigotted after 72 h and the patient allowed home.

Prophylactic antibiotics are unnecessary, but urine cultures should be checked weekly until the stent is removed after 6 weeks. Follow-up diuretic urography and renography should be performed 3 months after the procedure.

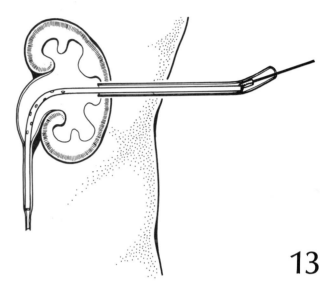

13

References

1. Wickham JEA, Kellett MJ. Percutaneous pyelolysis. *Eur Urol* 1983; 9: 122–4.

2. Whitfield HN, Mills V, Miller RA, Wickham JEA. Percutaneous pyelolysis: an alternative to pyeloplasty. *Br J Urol* 1983; Supplement: 93–6.

3. Davis DM. The process of ureteral repair: a recapitulation of the splinting question. *J Urol* 1958; 79: 215–23.

Transitional cell tumours

H. N. Whitfield MA, MChir, FRCS
Consultant Urologist, St Bartholomew's Hospital and St Mark's Hospital for Diseases of the Colon and Rectum, London, UK

Principles and justification

Indications

Opinion is divided as to whether a percutaneous approach to renal pelvic tumours is to be recommended. There has always been some reluctance to perform a radical nephroureterectomy for a solitary low-grade renal pelvic tumour. The risk exists, however, that during the dilatation of a nephrostomy track, intravascular dissemination of tumour cells could occur, particularly if the nephrostomy track is established through the tumour-bearing calix[1-3].

Preoperative

The diagnosis must have been made by combination of radiological, endoscopic and cytological criteria. The differentiation between a filling defect due to a transitional cell tumour and a non-opaque uric acid stone may be made by computed tomography.

Operation

A nephrostomy track is dilated though an appropriate calix to 30 Fr (*see* chapter on pp. 40–45).

The tumour may be removed by cold-cup biopsy forceps or using a resectoscope. The tumour base should be treated with diathermy.

Postoperative care

If adequate haemostasis has been secured, a JJ stent is not necessary, but a nephrostomy tube should be left *in situ* for 24–48 h.

Some authors advocate leaving a radioactive iridium wire in the nephrostomy tube to deliver 4500 cGy to the track[4].

Complications

The number of cases that have been treated in this way is too small to assess the potential for tumour recurrences in the renal pelvis or elsewhere.

References

1. Orihuela E, Smith AD. Percutaneous treatment of transitional cell carcinoma of the upper urinary tract. *Urol Clin North Am* 1988; 15: 425–31.

2. Smith AD, Orihuela E, Crowley AR. Percutaneous management of renal pelvic tumours: a treatment option in selected cases. *J Urol* 1987; 137: 852–6.

3. Tasca A, Zattoni F. The case of a percutaneous approach to transitional cell carcinoma of the renal pelvis. *J Urol* 1990; 143: 902–5.

4. Woodhouse CRJ, Kellett MJ, Bloom HJG. Percutaneous renal surgery and local radiotherapy in the management of renal pelvic transitional cell carcinoma. *Br J Urol* 1986; 58: 245–9.

Illustrations by Paul Richardson

Ureteroscopy

Demetrius H. Bagley MD
Department of Urology, Jefferson Medical College, Thomas Jefferson University, Philadelphia, Pennsylvania, USA

History

Ureteroscopy has rapidly become an important urological procedure with the development of new instruments and techniques. Although the first ureteroscopies were performed with flexible endoscopes, the rigid techniques, originally performed with paediatric instruments in women and later in both sexes with specially designed instruments, rapidly became predominant because of their practical application, particularly for ureteric calculi. As rigid ureteroscopes grew in length, the endoscopic reach of the urologist extended from the distal ureter to the mid and proximal ureter and even to the renal pelvis. The difficulty in passing these rigid instruments to the proximal sites also became apparent. Interest and technical developments again combined to produce flexible ureteroscopes with mechanisms for active deflection and with adequate working channels. With these instruments, the entire upper collecting system, including the intrarenal portion, have become accessible.

Principles and justification

Indications

As experience with ureteroscopy has increased, multiple indications for endoscopy of the upper urinary tract have been established. The diagnostic indications include filling defects, ureteric obstruction from an intrinsic filling defect, unilateral gross haematuria and abnormal urine cytology. The major therapeutic application has been for the removal of urinary calculi. Other indications have been the removal of foreign bodies, bypassing sites of obstruction or fistulae, ablation of bleeding lesions and treatment of low-grade upper tract neoplasms.

Contraindications

The major contraindication to ureteroscopy is the presence of an active urinary tract infection. However, even this may be only a relative contraindication since obstruction in the presence of an infection may be a major causative factor and may require endoscopic intervention for removal. There are other relative contraindications such as previous surgical intervention or anatomical abnormalities of the ureter which can be overcome.

Instruments

Ureteroscopes can be divided into three broad categories: the conventional or larger diameter rigid endoscope; the small-diameter rigid ureteroscope; and the flexible endoscopes. These instruments vary in size, optical systems and working or irrigating capacities. Therefore, each type is considered separately.

1 The standard or conventional ureteroscope, the earliest design, is similar to a cystoscope with interchangeable sheaths and rod lenses.

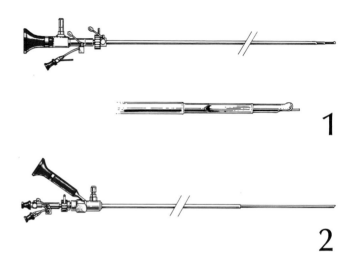

2 The working ureteroscopes have an offset eyepiece to allow insertion of a straight rigid ultrasound probe. Endoscopes with an integral telescope constructed as a one-piece instrument or an interchangeable sheath/telescope design are available. Although most endoscopes in this category have a rod lens system, at least two include a fibreoptic viewing system, giving flexibility to the offset ocular mount.

The small-diameter rigid ureteroscopes include those with a dimension of 8.5 Fr or less. These instruments were originally designed for use in the distal ureter but some are long enough to pass to the renal pelvis in certain patients. Most of these endoscopes have a fibreoptic viewing system and may possess one or two working channels. The small diameter usually permits their passage into the ureter without prior dilatation.

3 Flexible ureteroscopes can be divided into two groups: the actively and the passively deflectable endoscopes. The passively deflectable design possesses no mechanism for changing the direction of the tip and is of only limited clinical value. The actively deflectable instruments possess an intrinsic mechanism for changing the direction of the tip of the endoscope. These instruments are long enough to reach the renal pelvis and can potentially be passed into the intrarenal collecting system. They range in size from 8.5 to 10.2 Fr. The working channel is generally 3.6 Fr, although in the 8.5 Fr instrument it is 2.5 Fr. All of the flexible endoscopes have a fibreoptic optical system. Numerous flexible working instruments are available in sizes of 1.9–4.5 Fr. The individual design of these instruments will be considered in subsequent chapters.

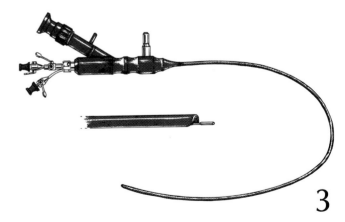

Preoperative

Anaesthesia

All types of anaesthesia have been used for uretero-scopy. Local anaesthesia with intravenous sedation monitored by an anaesthetist can be used for many simpler ureteroscopies, including distal stone removal and diagnostic flexible ureteroscopy as well as for treatment of some proximally located stones. General anaesthesia is preferable if a prolonged procedure is likely and when combined with other procedures, such as percutaneous nephrostomy. Spinal or epidural anaesthesia is effective, although the level must be quite high for intrarenal manipulation. It is often reserved for those patients in whom general anaesthesia is con-traindicated because of the patient's medical condition.

Operation

Position of patient

4 Patients may be placed in a standard lithotomy position: it is helpful to abduct the contralateral leg slightly. This position is convenient for standard cystoscopy and gives the urologist sufficient room to position the ureteroscope into even a laterally located orifice. Flexible ureteroscopy may be performed in the supine position or even with the patient prone and legs spread to give access to the urethra in the male or female.

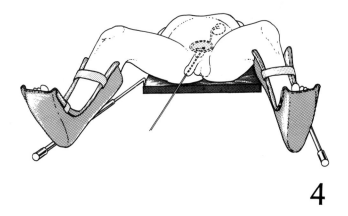

4

Ureteric dilatation

Demonstration that the ureterovesical junction could be satisfactorily dilated without significant permanent injury was one of the major steps in developing the techniques of ureteroscopy. Although the need for ureteric dilatation is now less because of the use of smaller endoscopes, it remains an important step in many ureteroscopic procedures.

The intramural portion of the ureter must be dilated if the lumen is too small to accept the endoscope used. It must often be dilated for the conventional rigid ureteroscopes and should be dilated to approximately 2 Fr larger than the shaft of the ureteroscope. Dilatation may also be used to extract some stones and to avoid lithotripsy.

Considerable discussion of ureteroscopy without ureteral dilatation has occurred. This can be achieved, particularly with smaller diameter endoscopes, but the normal ureteric orifice, which is approximately 3 mm in diameter, must be enlarged to accept a 12 Fr (or 4 mm) or larger endoscope. Some authors pass these endo-scopes without prior dilatation, clearly using the endoscope itself for dilatation.

Several techniques for ureteric dilatation have been employed, which include the use of a ureteric catheter or stent for passive dilatation of the ureter or acute techniques of active dilatation, including the use of graduated dilators or balloon dilating catheters.

5 A standard ureteric catheter placed into the ureter will effectively dilate the lumen and should be left in place for 12–24 h for effective dilatation. This was the first technique used for dilatation for ureteroscopy. Because of the time involved, it is now rarely used just for dilatation; however, when a catheter is placed for other purposes, such as for drainage of an obstructed ureter proximal to a calculus, subsequent ureteroscopy can usually be performed without any further dilatation.

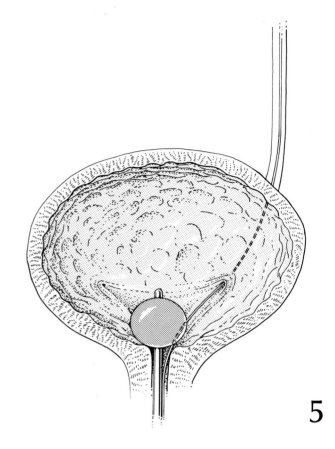

5

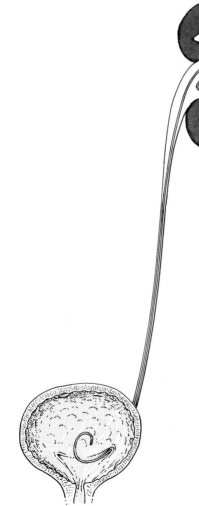

6

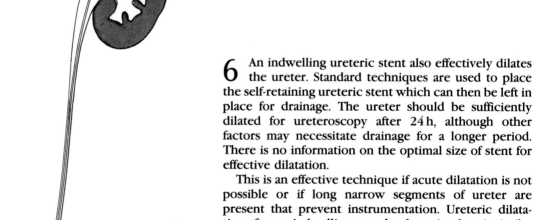

6 An indwelling ureteric stent also effectively dilates the ureter. Standard techniques are used to place the self-retaining ureteric stent which can then be left in place for drainage. The ureter should be sufficiently dilated for ureteroscopy after 24 h, although other factors may necessitate drainage for a longer period. There is no information on the optimal size of stent for effective dilatation.

This is an effective technique if acute dilatation is not possible or if long narrow segments of ureter are present that prevent instrumentation. Ureteric dilatation after an indwelling stent has been in place is similar to that seen with a ureteric catheter. The entire length of the ureter is dilated to an extent that is usually adequate to accept even the larger (13 Fr) rigid ureteroscopes.

7 Graduated tapered semi-rigid dilators offer a convenient, inexpensive technique for acute dilatation of the ureterovesical junction. To dilate the ureter a guidewire is placed cystoscopically. The dilators are then passed sequentially over the guidewire, and should be advanced approximately 6–8 cm to ensure that they are passing through the intramural portion of the ureter. Usually a 6-Fr or 8-Fr dilator is used initially. Each is passed into the distal ureter and then removed. The larger dilators (12–14 Fr) may not fit through the working port of the cystoscope and must therefore be passed over the wire and followed fluoroscopically. The sheath of the cystoscope should be left in place to stabilize the dilator in its course through the urethra and bladder. It is usually quite easy to pass the dilators from 6 Fr to approximately 12 Fr but larger dilators (14 or 16 Fr) are considerably more difficult.

Other graduated dilators are available that increase in size from 6 to 12 Fr or 10 to 18 Fr and ensure that the lumen can be dilated to 12 Fr with passage of a single instrument: it can be dilated further to 18 Fr with passage of a single second instrument.

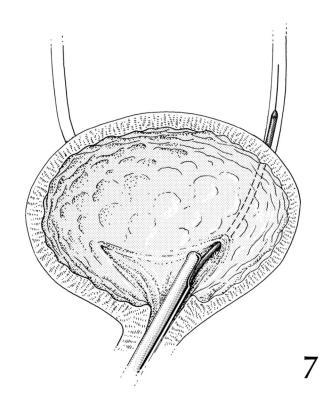

7

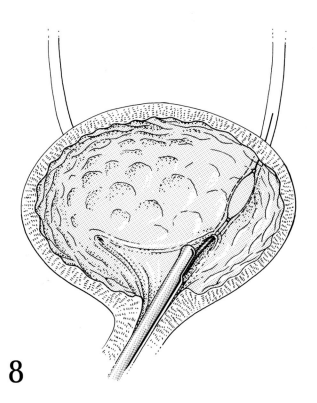

8

8 Olive-tipped metal bougies can also be used for dilatation, and can be passed over a guidewire in a fashion similar to the graduated dilators. They should be passed through the intramural portion of the ureter to ensure full dilatation. Increasing sizes are passed sequentially, also to ensure full dilatation. The larger sizes (such as 12 or 14 Fr) may not fit through the working port of the cystoscope, and it is often necessary to remove the bridge and telescope, place the dilators over the guidewire and then pass the handle in a retrograde fashion through the bridge as the cystoscope is reassembled.

9 Balloon dilating catheters offer a convenient and effective technique for dilatation at any level in the ureter. Several different sizes of balloons are available; the usual sizes employed are 15 and 18 Fr, which offer adequate dilatation without ureteric damage.

To use a balloon dilating catheter a guidewire is first placed cystoscopically. The balloon catheter is then advanced over the guidewire and the balloon is placed to give full dilatation of the desired region. The balloon tapers at each end and the cylindrical portion should be at the desired point for full dilatation: for example, to dilate the ureterovesical junction the cylindrical portion of the balloon should extend from the ureteric orifice proximally through the intramural portion of the ureter. Balloons designed specifically for dilatation expand to a certain fixed diameter with increasing pressure until they reach the point of rupture. In contrast, balloons constructed of elastic materials (such as latex) continue to expand until they fracture: latex balloons should *not* be used for dilatation as they will not dilate a narrow segment but rather will stay small in that area and balloon into a more pliable portion of the ureter.

To expand the balloon and dilate the ureter, the balloon is filled with a mixture of saline and contrast medium in sufficient concentration to demonstrate the balloon's presence fluoroscopically. The pressure in the balloon is then increased until any narrow segment or waist is fully expanded. The pressure should be monitored with an in-line gauge and should not exceed the manufacturer's recommended specifications. The balloon should then be deflated fully by aspirating the contrast-containing solution before the catheter is removed.

Other dilating balloons are available which will fit through a 5-Fr or even a 3.5-Fr lumen in a ureteroscope to dilate narrow segments under direct vision. These balloons are generally more fragile and cannot be inflated to as high a pressure as the standard balloons mounted on a 5-Fr or 7-Fr catheter.

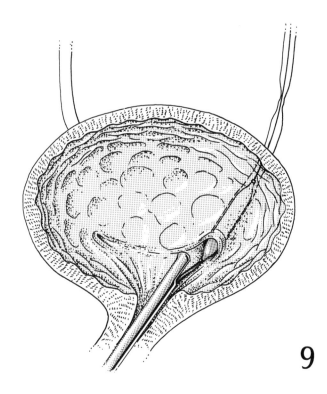

9

Irrigation

Irrigation is essential to clear the field of view and to distend the ureteric lumen. In general, the lowest pressure possible should be used to achieve these goals: when the irrigating or working channel is empty in any of the ureteroscopes, adequate irrigation can be achieved by gravity alone, but when the channel is filled some pressure system is needed to pass irrigant through the channel. The different systems developed include a manually powered syringe, a pressurized bag, and a pumping device.

The standard irrigant is normal saline. Some risk of absorption from perforation and extravasation or from pyelovenous backflow is present and therefore a sterile physiological solution must be used. Radiographic contrast may be added to the irrigant if needed to opacify the collecting system. For fulguration with monopolar electrosurgical instruments, a non-conducting solution such as glycine or water can be used for short periods, during which the intraluminal pressure can be followed clinically.

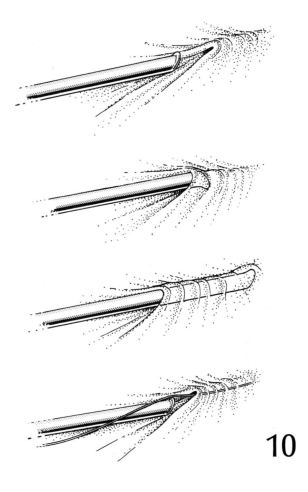

Passing a rigid ureteroscope into the ureter

10 The techniques of passing the endoscope into the ureter vary with the ureteroscope employed. The small diameter ureteroscopes can be placed under direct vision into the ureter, usually without prior dilatation but dilatation is usually necessary for the larger endoscopes. The intramural portion of the ureter may seem tight but as long as the lumen can be visualized the instrument can be advanced and used to dilate the lumen: if the lumen is not visible, the instrument should not be advanced. A guidewire or a ureteric catheter placed through the working channel of the ureteroscope into the ureter can be used as a guide to the lumen.

Most rigid ureteroscopes are tapered or graduated so that the more proximal shaft of the instrument will dilate the distal ureter.

10

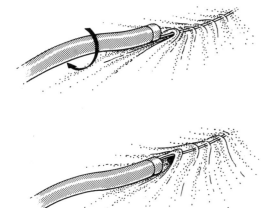

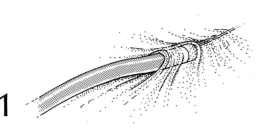

Inserting the flexible ureteroscope

11 Direct insertion of the flexible ureteroscope is often difficult because of the instability imposed by its flexibility, if the orifice is obscured by blood, and also because of the narrow field of view. The instrument may coil in the bladder as it meets resistance to passing into the ureteric orifice.

11

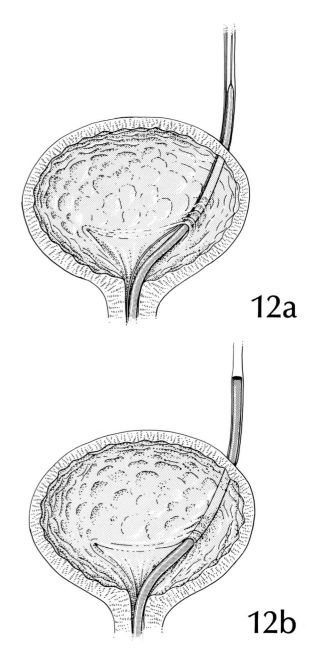

12a, b The flexible ureteroscope may be stabilized for passage into the ureter by introducing a flexible guide tube on a graduated dilator. The dilator is then removed, leaving the lumen of the sheath available from the meatus through the urethra and bladder into the ureter. However, difficulties with this technique are kinking of the sheath in the male urethra, presence of a blood clot or impingement of the mucosa on the tip of the sheath, or damage to the ureter from the tip of the sheath. The technique is most useful in patients when the ureteroscope must be removed and inserted repeatedly (as for fragmentation and removal of a large calculus, particularly in women).

The most satisfactory technique for insertion of the flexible ureteroscope is generally with the use of a guidewire. Two guidewires may be placed cystoscopically for any manipulative procedure, or a single guidewire placed for a simple observational diagnostic procedure. The ureterovesical junction is then dilated to 2 Fr sizes larger than the shaft of the ureteroscope. The cystoscope is removed, and one guidewire is clipped to the drapes as a safety while the other is used as the working wire. The working wire is placed into the channel of the ureteroscope and an assistant holds the guidewire as the endoscope is advanced with fluoroscopic monitoring of its position in the same way as an open end ureteric catheter. Care must be taken to orientate the tip of the ureteroscope at the orifice to allow the guidewire to lift the orifice and facilitate entry of the endoscope. The guidewire is necessary for stabilization only until the endoscope reaches above the level of the iliac vessels.

There may be several reasons why the ureteroscope does not pass proximal portions of the ureter. A narrow segment may not admit the endoscope, but this can often be determined with endoscopic visualization of the area and if necessary that area can be dilated with a balloon or graduated dilator. The balloon catheter may be of the type passed over a guidewire and positioned fluoroscopically or may be small and passed through the lumen of the ureteroscope to dilate the segment under direct vision.

Sufficient friction between a flexible ureteroscope and the wall of the ureter may occur to prevent its advancement, causing the ureteroscope to coil in the bladder. This problem can be alleviated by placing a guidewire through the ureteroscope to stiffen the more proximal portion which passes through the bladder and the distal ureter.

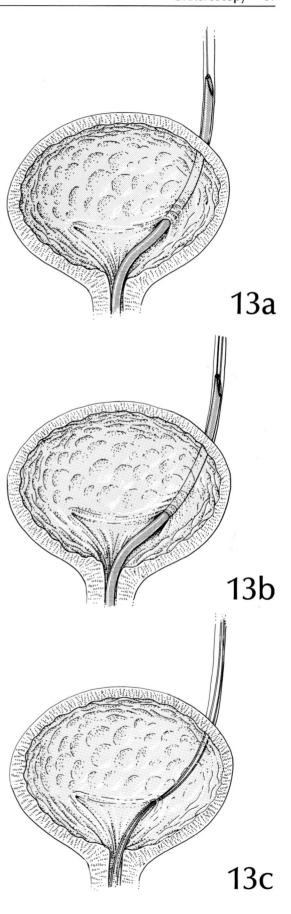

13a

13a–c If the ureteroscope is removed and then needs to be reinserted but the channel is occupied by a working instrument, another working wire must be placed. Either a dilator sheath system or a double lumen catheter is placed over the safety guidewire and advanced into the distal or mid ureter under fluoroscopic control. The additional guidewire is then placed through the sheath or catheter into the ureter. The safety wire is then again clipped to the drape and the new working wire used for reinserting the ureteroscope.

13b

13c

Postoperative care

A major factor affecting the patient's postoperative course seems to be oedema at the level of ureteric dilatation or manipulation. Intraluminal drainage is necessary in these patients, using either an indwelling ureteric catheter or a self-retaining ureteric stent. A catheter is usually left in place for 24–48 h, judged by clearing of any haematuria; a self-retaining stent, such as a double-pigtail stent, is left in place until the patient returns for a follow-up visit (usually at 1–2 weeks). The stent can then be removed using a flexible cystoscope, or with a urethral string if a 'dangler' type of stent was used. The ureteric catheter gives excellent control and allows the quality of urinary output to be monitored but does require hospitalization for a short period. The self-retaining stent allows earlier discharge but often causes irritation and must be removed in a second interventional procedure.

Patients are examined 1–2 weeks after the procedure for urinalysis and to follow their symptoms, and again 6–8 weeks later for renal ultrasonography to identify any postoperative ureteric obstruction. Subsequent follow up depends on the disease process.

Further reading

Bagley DH. Removal of upper urinary calculi with flexible ureteropyeloscopy. *Urology* 1990; 35: 412–16.

Bagley DH (ed.). *Techniques with the Flexible Ureteroscope.* Stamford: Circon-ACMI, 1991.

Bagley DH, Allen J. Flexible ureteropyeloscopy in the diagnosis of benign essential hematuria. *J Urol* 1990; 143: 549–53.

Bagley DH, Huffman JL, Lyon ES. Flexible ureteropyeloscopy: diagnosis and treatment in the upper urinary tract. *J Urol* 1987; 138: 280–5.

Dretler SP, Watson G, Parrish JA, Murray S. Pulsed dye laser fragmentation of ureteral calculi: initial clinical experience. *J Urol* 1987; 137: 386–9.

Huffman JL, Bagley DH, Lyon ES (eds). *Ureteroscopy.* Philadelphia: WB Saunders, 1987.

Huffman JL, Bagley DH, Schoenberg HW, Lyon ES. Transurethral removal of large ureteral and renal pelvic calculi using ureteroscopic ultrasonic lithotripsy. *J Urol* 1983; 130: 31–4.

Kavoussi L, Clayman RV, Basler JW. Flexible actively deflectable fiberoptic ureteronephroscopy. *J Urol* 1989; 142: 949–54.

Lyon ES, Banno JJ, Schoenberg HW. Transurethral ureteroscopy in men using juvenile cystoscopy equipment. *J Urol* 1979; 122: 152–3.

Seeger AR, Rittenberg MH, Bagley DH. Ureteropyeloscopic removal of ureteral calculi. *J Urol* 1988; 139: 1180–3.

Thomas R. Rigid ureteroscopy: pitfalls and remedies. *Urology* 1988; 32: 328–34.

Ureteroscopy for non-calculous applications

Demetrius H. Bagley MD
Department of Urology, Jefferson Medical College, Thomas Jefferson University, Philadelphia, Pennsylvania, USA

Ureteroscopy has many applications for diagnosis and treatment besides its major use for removing calculi: endoscopic observation alone can be a very important diagnostic procedure. The addition of working instruments capable of sampling tissue has expanded the diagnostic applications further.

Instruments

Endoscopes

1 The same ureteroscopes as are used for other procedures can be employed for non-calculous indications. A rigid endoscopic resectoscope similar to the larger standard transurethral resectoscopes may be used for removing neoplasms accessible to a rigid endoscope.

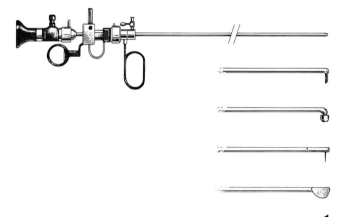

1

Working devices

$2a, b$ Several designs of cup forceps are available to sample tissue ureteroscopically, down to as small as 3 Fr. The sample obtained from any of these is quite small and is often best handled by cytological techniques. Grasping devices, such as baskets or wire-pronged graspers, can be used to remove relatively large volumes of friable neoplasms. These are available in a wide range of sizes.

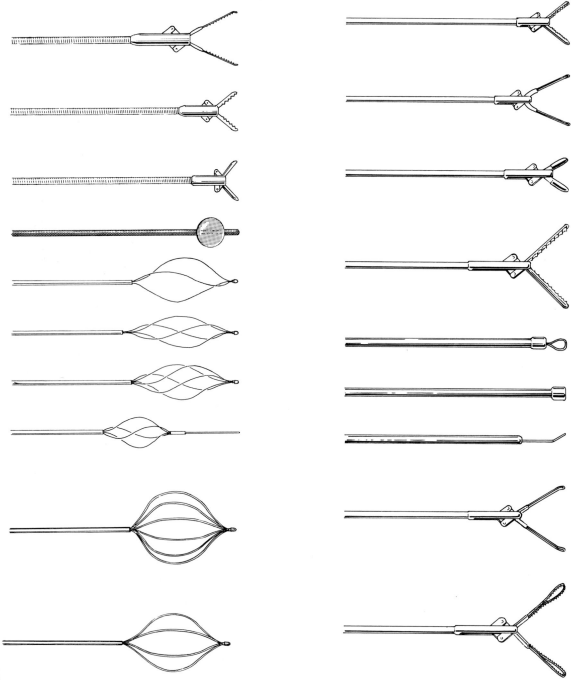

2a

2b

Procedures

EVALUATION AND TREATMENT OF UPPER TRACT FILLING DEFECTS

3, 4 The most valuable differential diagnostic procedure for the evaluation of upper tract filling defects is endoscopic observation. The typical granular appearance of the calculus (*Illustration 3*) can be distinguished easily from the tissue of a neoplasm (*Illustration 4*). A neoplasm is observed by passing the ureteroscope to the level of the filling defect. Contrast used in the irrigant can demonstrate fluoroscopically the position of the endoscope and collecting system and confirm that the instrument is at the lesion in question. Irrigation should be continued as necessary to clear the field of view to allow adequate observation.

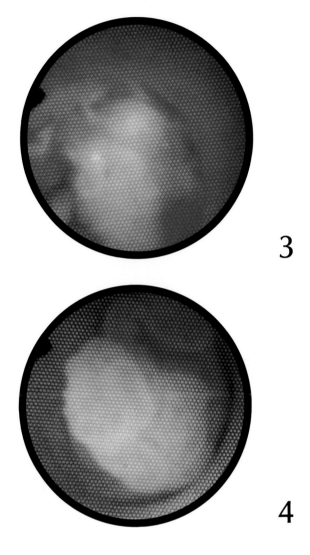

3

4

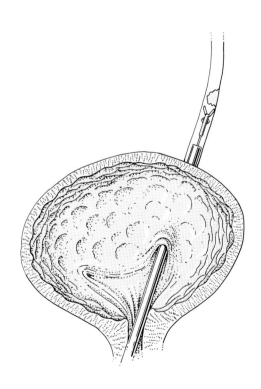

5

5 Any lesion suspicious of a neoplasm should be biopsied; a cup biopsy forceps will obtain a piece of tissue satisfactory for diagnosis. The cup forceps is passed through the endoscope to the central base of the lesion, closed and then removed with the sample. If there is no adherent tissue extending beyond the cup, the forceps can be withdrawn through the working channel. If, however, tumour extends beyond the cup, the larger piece can be obtained as a sample only if the entire unit (ureteroscope, forceps and tumour) is removed intact, which will necessitate replacement of the ureteroscope.

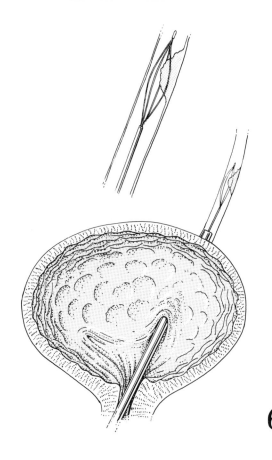

6a

6a, b Other devices give very satisfactory tissue samples. A basket, particularly a double snare design, will remove a large piece of friable tumour, such as a low-grade transitional cell carcinoma. The basket should be placed through the working channel, opened, pressed onto the friable tumour and partially closed. It is then withdrawn from the tumour, dragging with it a relatively large sample of the neoplasm. Lesions up to 1 cm may be removed in this way. Again, the entire unit of ureteroscope, basket and sample should be removed to avoid shearing the sample off by withdrawing the basket into the ureteroscope. Helical baskets and wire pronged graspers may be used similarly.

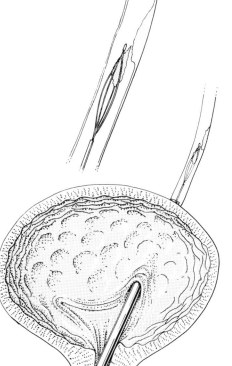

6b

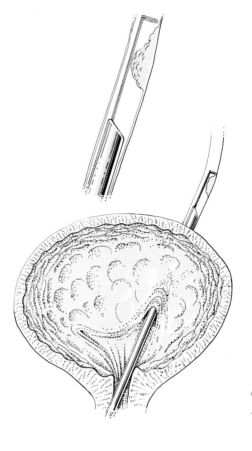

7a

7a, b The ureteric resectoscope can be employed in an area accessible to a rigid ureteroscope. The loop is passed beyond the tumour and used to draw the fronds of tumour into the sheath. A fulgurating current is then applied to cut the tumour and fulgurate the base. One sample usually must be removed from the ureteroscope before the next sample is taken. Resection should be continued only to the wall of the ureter and not through it, as it is very thin.

After sampling and removal of most of the volume of small neoplasms, the base of the remaining tumour can be fulgurated with an electrode, usually 3 Fr. Alternatively, an NdYAG laser can be used, which is usually activated at 15 W and applied to the lesion until it is coagulated to a whitish appearance. To avoid stricture, fulguration should be limited to less than half the circumference of the ureter and should be performed as superficially as possible.

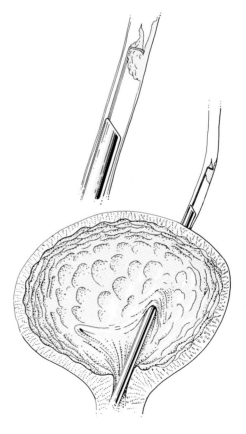

7b

EVALUATION AND TREATMENT IN PATIENTS WITH GROSS UNILATERAL HAEMATURIA

Small haemangiomas and minute venous ruptures were the most common lesions seen in a series of patients studied by ureteroscopy[1]. Haemangiomas appear as typical erythematous raised lesions usually on a papilla. These small lesions can be treated directly by fulguration with a 2-Fr or 3-Fr electrode or a NdYAG laser. If there is any question regarding the nature of the lesion, a biopsy may be performed with a cup forceps. However, bleeding may be brisk and fulguration without previous biopsy is preferred.

The entire mucosa of the upper collecting system should be observed in patients with gross unilateral haematuria. This is best performed using a combination of a small-diameter rigid ureteroscope to observe the distal ureter without prior dilatation and an actively deflectable, flexible ureteroscope to observe the mid and upper ureter and intrarenal collecting system. With this combined approach, the entire mucosa can be observed without prior instrumentation of the surface. Initially after cystoscopy, a small-diameter rigid ureteroscope is placed transurethrally and passed into the ureteric orifice. The circumference of the lumen should be observed to the extent of the range of the rigid endoscope, usually at the level of the iliac vessels but possibly extending to the proximal ureter. A guidewire is left in place to the mid-ureter as the rigid ureteroscope is removed. The ureterovesical junction can then be dilated as necessary and a flexible ureteroscope placed over the guidewire to the point previously observed by the rigid endoscope. The mucosa is then observed with the flexible endoscope as it is passed proximally within the ureter. The renal pelvis is observed next and then the individual infundibula and calices, passing systematically from the upper pole through the mid and lower portions of the collecting system. Most lesions have been seen on papillae or in the calices and these areas should be studied meticulously.

REMOVAL OF PROXIMALLY LOCATED INDWELLING STENTS

The tip of a self-retaining ureteric stent may withdraw into the ureteric orifice or may be badly positioned initially: in either case, the stent is not retrievable by simple cystoscopy alone. These stents may be reached ureteroscopically. Those in the distal ureter may be approached with a rigid ureteroscope while stents in the proximal ureter or entirely in the renal pelvis may be removed with a flexible ureteroscope. It is usually possible to see the stent although placing a retrieval device around its tip may be difficult: a three-pronged grasper may be useful for grasping the stent. Stiffer stents made of material such as polyurethane may be too firm to hold with a wire-pronged grasper; in these cases a basket placed over the end of the stent will hold it for retrieval. The ureter is usually already dilated and further dilatation is unnecessary either to place the ureteroscope or to remove the stent.

References

1. Bagley DH. Flexible ureteropyeloscopy in the diagnosis of benign essential hematuria. *J Urol* 1990; 143: 549–53.

Ureteroscopic treatment of upper urinary tract calculi

Demetrius H. Bagley MD
Department of Urology, Jefferson Medical College, Thomas Jefferson University, Philadelphia, Pennsylvania, USA

History

The endoscopic treatment of ureteric and renal calculi has progressed rapidly over a 10-year period. Early attempts were limited by the size of calculi and the capability of retrieval alone. With the development of appropriate working ureteroscopes, small ultrasound probes, electrohydraulic lithotriptor probes and pulsed-dye lasers, endoscopic lithotripsy has become a reality for all but extremely large stones. The advent of extracorporeal shock wave lithotripsy gave another avenue of treatment for some of the smaller, simpler stones; endoscopy remains for the more complicated situations.

Principles and justification

Indications

Any ureteric calculus may be approached ureteroscopically. Most upper ureteric calculi are treated preferentially with shock wave lithotripsy, but mid-ureteric stones which cannot be seen on ultrasonography or with fluoroscopy may be treated with ureteroscopy. Stones in the distal ureter are treated ureteroscopically with a very high success rate; shock wave lithotripsy has an acceptable but lower success rate. Stones in the upper urinary tract which have been unsuccessfully treated with shock wave lithotripsy may be treated endoscopically. Most large renal calculi are treated effectively by a percutaneous approach, while most large ureteric stones may be more successfully removed with a ureteroscopic approach.

Instruments

Endoscopes

Any of the endoscopes discussed in the chapter on ureteroscopy (pp. 53–62) can be employed for the removal of calculi. The working instrument must be matched to the appropriate ureteroscope. For example, 4.5-Fr flexible devices will fit through the working channel of many large conventional ureteroscopes but will not fit any of the smaller diameter rigid or flexible ureteroscopes.

Numerous grasping devices are available, ranging in size from 1.9. to 4.5 Fr for use through the wide variety of endoscopes available. Grasping devices include helical baskets, double snare (Segura) baskets, single snares, two- three- and four-pronged wire graspers, and various styled forceps.

Lithotripters

Ultrasonic lithotripter

Ultrasonic lithotripsy can be used effectively for fragmenting ureteric calculi. The small-diameter rigid probes must be passed through a straight channel, and therefore a rigid ureteroscope with an offset eyepiece must be used. Both rigid and hollow-probe designs are available. The hollow probes will remove some of the smaller fragments while the rigid probes are more powerful and give more rapid fragmentation. These can not be used through flexible endoscopes. The ultrasound probe must be applied directly to the calculus for fragmentation.

Electrohydraulic lithotripter

For electrohydraulic lithotripsy a high-voltage discharge is applied across a coaxial tip of a probe. When this occurs within a fluid medium, a bubble is formed which rapidly contracts, setting up shock waves within the medium, which will set up stresses within the crystalline structure of an adjacent calculus, and cause it to fragment. Probe sizes available range from 1.6 to 9.0 Fr. The history of use of the electrohydraulic lithotripter in the bladder is long; it has also proved safe and effective in the ureter and intrarenal collecting system.

Laser lithotripter

The pulsed-dye laser is the most widely applied and most effective laser for lithotripsy. Pulsed light of 504 nm lasting 1–2 µs is carried along quartz fibres 200–500 µm in diameter. The tip of the fibre must touch the calculus to initiate the photoacoustic effect which fragments the stone. This is a very controlled and safe technique but the instrument is considerably more expensive than the other lithotripters mentioned. The fibre may be passed through rigid or flexible endoscopes.

Operation

The approach differs depending on the location of the stone. Rigid endoscopes are the first choice for treating stones below the iliac vessels in the distal third of the ureter. The rigid endoscope can be manoeuvred into the ureter and allows placement of a basket or lithotripter device. In contrast, a flexible ureteroscope in the distal ureter tends to fall back into the bladder, necessitating reinsertion of the ureteroscope into the orifice.

1, 2a, b A small stone is usually easily retrieved. It is visualized (*Illustration 1*), a basket is placed under direct vision through the ureteroscope and the wires are placed around the calculus (*Illustration 2*).

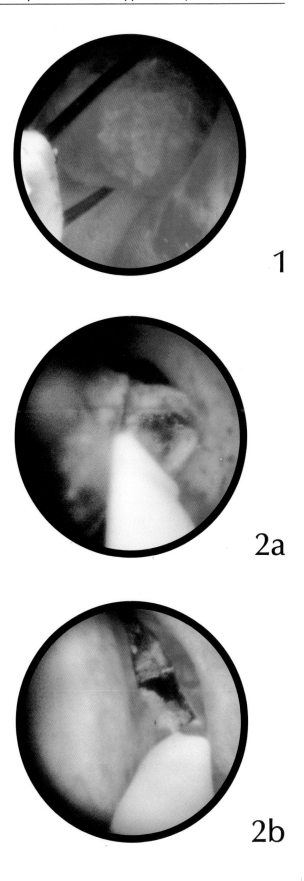

1

2a

2b

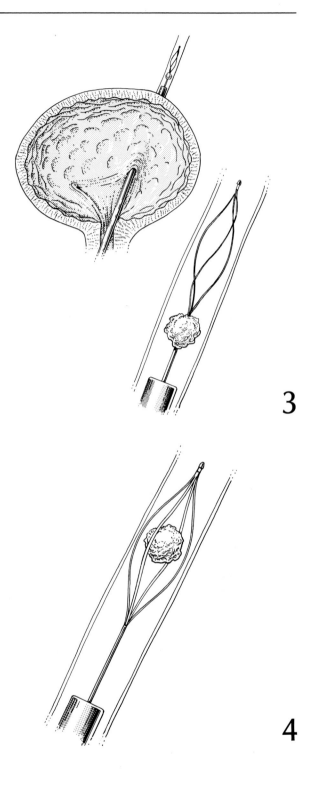

3

4

3,4 If there is little space around the calculus, a helical basket is more easily manipulated onto the stone. If the stone moves freely in the ureter and more space is available, a double snare basket can be placed to engage the stone more easily.

The basket is closed under vision while the urologist makes certain that no mucosa is trapped within the basket. The entire unit (stone, basket and ureteroscope) is then removed from the ureter. The urologist should observe the stone during removal to ensure that it does not become trapped in a narrow segment of the ureter.

Wire-pronged graspers may also be used for retrieving these stones but hold them less securely. However, wire-pronged graspers are particularly useful for smaller fragments that cannot be trapped easily in a basket.

More proximally located stones may also be approached with a rigid ureteroscope, although it is often easier to pass a flexible ureteroscope into the proximal ureter. If a rigid endoscope is successfully manoeuvred to the proximal ureter, the options of using basket or graspers are the same. There is only a single working channel available with a flexible ureteroscope and it is preferable to attempt to retrieve the stones with a reversible instrument such as a three-wire-pronged grasper. A stone that becomes lodged in a narrow portion of the ureter as the endoscope and calculus are withdrawn may be disengaged from the prongs of the grasper very easily. A lithotripter device may then be passed through the working channel to fragment the stone into retrievable pieces.

If a basket has been used to grasp the stone and becomes lodged in the ureter it may be impossible to disengage the stone and remove the basket. The handle of the basket must then be removed and the ureteroscope removed from the basket, leaving the stone and the basket within the ureter. The flexible ureteroscope

is reinserted adjacent to the shaft of the basket to fragment the stone into pieces that can be removed to allow removal of the basket.

Larger calculi must be broken into smaller pieces which can be removed through the lumen of the ureter. Three different lithotripters have been used successfully for treating ureteric stones.

ULTRASONIC LITHOTRIPSY

$5a, b$ Rigid ultrasonic lithotripter probes may be passed through a straight channel in a ureteroscope with an offset eyepiece. Impacted stones can be fragmented *in situ* (*Illustration 5a*) but freely moving stones should be engaged in a basket initially to prevent retrograde movement (*Illustration 5b*).

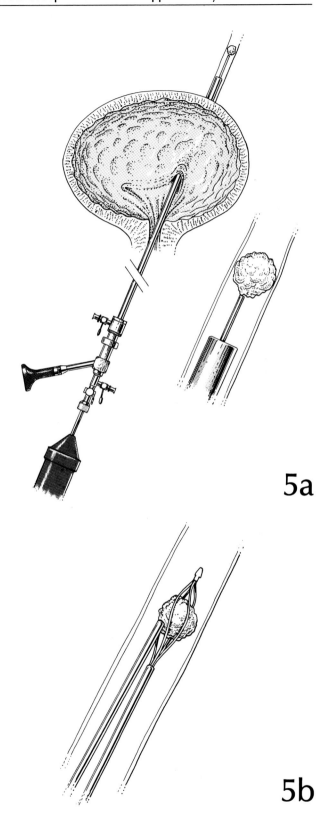

5a

5b

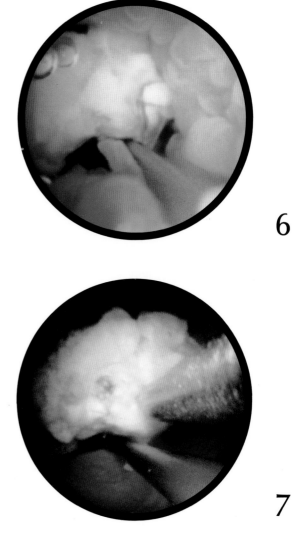

6

7

6,7 The calculus is secured in the basket and the ultrasound probe is passed through the working channel of the instrument and activated to fragment the stone. As lithotripsy continues fragments are aspirated through the hollow ultrasound probe. After removal of the major fragments, the ureteroscope is replaced to inspect the ureter and to remove any fragments over about 2 mm diameter.

ELECTROHYDRAULIC LITHOTRIPSY

Any of the ureteroscopes may be used to place an electrohydraulic lithotripter probe, depending upon the size available. Once the ureteroscope is placed in the ureter and the calculus is visualized, the electrohydraulic lithotripter probe is passed through the working channel and placed in approximation to the central portion of the calculus. It is then activated with single shocks to fragment the stone. Care should be taken to place the probe towards the centre of the stone away from the mucosa. Fragmentation continues until the pieces are small enough to be removed from the ureter.

Saline irrigation is generally adequate to support activation of the probe, but if the spark appears insufficient to fragment the stone, the irrigant should be changed to one-sixth normal saline, which may give a more effective spark.

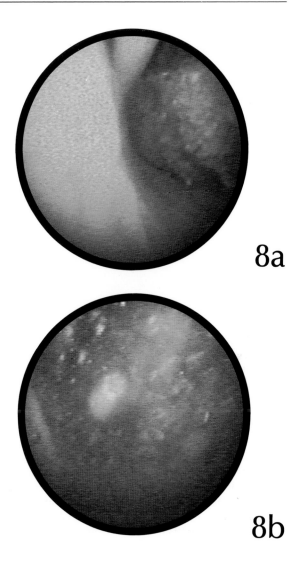

8a

8b

LASER LITHOTRIPSY

8a, b The laser light guide shows where the laser fibre is directed (*Illustration 8a*). When the laser is fired, stone fragments partially obscure vision. To ensure effective fragmentation the laser fibre must touch the calculus. The ureteroscope is inserted and the calculus visualized. The fibre is then passed through the working channel and applied to an irregular area or cleavage plane in the calculus and the pulsed-dye laser activated to fragment the stone. A relatively slow rate (3–5 Hz) is used initially, to minimize movement of the stone. The initial energy setting is related to the type of stone encountered. If the stone is the dark, smooth, typical calcium oxalate monohydrate, then the setting should be 80–100 mJ; a more fragile stone, such as a granular-appearing calcium oxalate dihydrate calculus, is usually fragmented with a lower setting (60–80 mJ). A stone which fragments quite easily can be broken into tiny fragments all of which can be allowed to pass, but a larger or more resistant stone should be broken into retrievable pieces.

Impacted calculus

Stones impacted in the ureter form a major portion of those presenting for endoscopic removal since they are less effectively treated by shock wave lithotripsy. These stones also present other problems, particularly because they often cannot be bypassed by a guidewire and therefore dilatation of the segment of the ureter below the stone may be difficult. Small-diameter rigid ureteroscopes are particularly useful for treatment of stones impacted in the distal ureter. The ureteroscope can be passed under direct vision and passed to the level of the calculus and a guidewire can be passed beyond the calculus under direct vision even if it will not pass cystoscopically. The calculus may be fragmented under direct vision with either the electrohydraulic lithotripter, by ultrasonic lithotripsy or by laser. If a small-diameter endoscope is not available, the distal ureter should be dilated initially with unguided metal dilators and the ureteroscope passed under direct vision. Lithotripsy can then be performed under vision.

Calculi impacted in the mid or proximal ureter may be approached with the flexible ureteroscope, passing the endoscope directly to the calculus. Fragmentation may then be started with the stone impacted, or a guidewire can be placed adjacent to the stone under direct vision.

Postoperative care

After any but the simplest stone removal, the ureter and kidney should be drained intraluminally with a catheter or stent. A plain abdominal radiograph showing kidneys, ureters and bladder (KUB) is taken after surgery in order to assess any residual stone fragments before catheter removal. Prophylactic antibiotics should be administered for 24–72 h after the procedure.

Ureteric catheterization

David A. Tolley FRCS, FRCS(Ed)
Director, Scottish Lithotriptor Centre and Consultant Urological Surgeon, Western General Hospital, Edinburgh, UK

Principles and justification

Ureteric catheters are used principally for evaluation and diagnosis of upper urinary tract abnormalities. Retrograde injection of radio-opaque contrast medium allows evaluation of upper urinary tract filling defects, and aspiration of urine from a ureteric catheter enables exfoliative cytological examination to be performed.

They may also be used for retrograde manipulation of ureteric stones, for temporary relief of ureteric obstruction, and as temporary stents following ureteric instrumentation or perforation.

The choice of ureteric catheter will depend on the purpose for which the catheter is required.

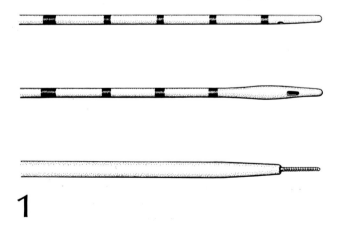

1 For diagnostic radiological examination of the renal pelvis and the calices, a 4-Fr or 5-Fr standard ureteric catheter is used, but for retrograde ureterography the use of an olivary-tipped catheter (Brasch or Chevassu) is recommended.

For retrograde stone manipulation, the largest possible size of catheter should be used, up to 8-Fr diameter. Alternatively, an open tipped 8-Fr or 9-Fr polyethylene catheter inserted over a guidewire may be used.

Temporary drainage of the upper urinary tract can be achieved using any size of catheter, but it should be borne in mind that small flexible catheters are more comfortable than larger rigid ones.

Operation

A cystoscopy is performed and the ureteric orifice is identified. A visual estimate of the size of the orifice is made, and an appropriate size of ureteric catheter is chosen.

2 An operating bridge or an Albarran deflector is used, and the catheter is inserted through the rubber bung of this attachment with the stylet in place.

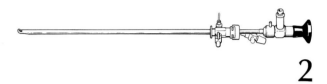

2

Once the tip of the catheter is visualized, the cystoscope is moved towards the ureteric orifice.

When catheterization is performed for ureteric drainage, the catheter containing its stylet is gently passed into the ureter up to the first mark on the catheter, i.e. 1 cm. The tip of the catheter now lies beyond the ureterovesical junction.

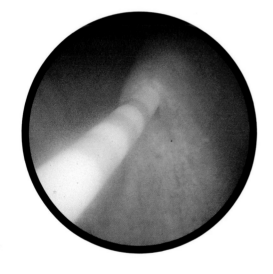

3

3 The stylet is withdrawn, and the catheter advanced as far as is necessary, as judged by fluoroscopy or by the marks on the catheter. Catheters are marked at 1-cm intervals by a single bar and at 5-cm intervals by multiple bars, e.g. three bars correspond to 15 cm. It is normally sufficient to advance the catheter to the fifth multiple mark, i.e. 25 cm, to be certain that it lies in the renal pelvis.

4 If a radiographic study of the renal pelvis and calices is to be undertaken, retrograde pyelography is performed. Once the catheter is visualized within the bladder, the stylet is withdrawn, and contrast medium is injected through the catheter until bubbling stops. This ensures that the ureteric catheter is free of air bubbles that could be mistaken for filling defects in the collecting system if injected with the contrast medium. The catheter is then introduced through the ureteric orifice and advanced for 25 cm; 5 ml of contrast medium is injected during radiographic screening of the coned area and radiographs taken as required.

If the whole length of the ureter is to be examined, ascending ureterography is required. Following elimination of air, the tip of the catheter is firmly placed into the ureteric orifice and up to 20 ml contrast medium is injected during fluoroscopic screening to outline the whole of the upper urinary tract.

Once the diagnostic procedure is complete, the ureteric catheter is withdrawn with the cystoscope. If the catheter is to remain in place temporarily, however, the Albarran bridge insert is partly withdrawn from the cystoscope sheath, and the ureteric catheter is grasped between thumb and forefinger once it becomes visible

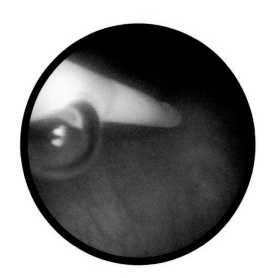

4

within the cystoscope sheath. This enables the movable bridge and telescope to be removed without dislodging the ureteric catheter. The cystoscope sheath is then gently removed while exerting mild counter-pressure on the ureteric catheter.

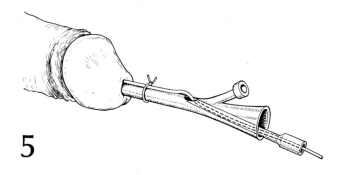

5

5 A latex foam catheter is inserted into the bladder, to which the ureteric catheter may be secured with tape or a suture.

Further stability can be obtained by inserting the ureteric catheter into the lumen of the urethral catheter through a wide-bore needle; alternatively, it may drain separately into a drainage bag.

Illustrations by Peter Cox

Placement of ureteric stents

David A. Tolley FRCS, FRCS(Ed)
Director, Scottish Lithotriptor Centre and Consultant Urological Surgeon, Western General Hospital,
Edinburgh, UK

History

Short-term and long-term drainage of the urinary tract may be achieved by stenting. Early stents were made of polyethylene and were generally inserted at open surgery. Endoscopic placement was first reported in 1967[1].

Modifications of catheter design, materials and methods of insertion have occurred since the first description of the use of a pigtail catheter placed cystoscopically in 1978 and the description of a JJ flexible silicone catheter by Finney in the same year [2, 3].

Ureteric stents are used in conjunction with renal stone management to relieve ureteric or ureteropelvic junction obstruction or to bypass ureteric fistulae.

Principles and justification

Contraindications

1 There are few contraindications to the use of ureteric catheters or stents, but anatomical abnormalities such as gross ureteric distortion make stent placement difficult, and lack of access to the distal ureter in patients with ileal conduits or with gross prostatic hypertrophy may preclude retrograde ureteric catheterization. Long-term ureteric stenting with the same stent is contraindicated in patients with stone formation or in those receiving cancer chemotherapy, because of the increased risk of encrustation.

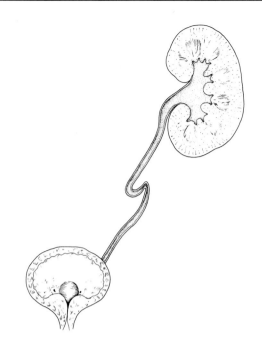

1

Preoperative

A plain abdominal radiograph and a recent intravenous urogram that clearly outlines the ureteric anatomy must be available before surgery. Alternatively, intraoperative ureterography should be carried out before stent placement.

Of equal importance is the choice of stent to be used. The choice of ureteric stents is bewildering. Most stents are made from silicone rubber or polyurethane; the latter are more rigid and must be used for antegrade stent placement. Much has been made of the non-irritant properties of silicone rubber, but controlled trials have failed to show any advantage for this type of material over the cheaper polyurethane stents in terms of encrustation. Some stents are now coated with a hydrophilic material, which becomes slippery when placed in contact with water, and this facilitates stent insertion.

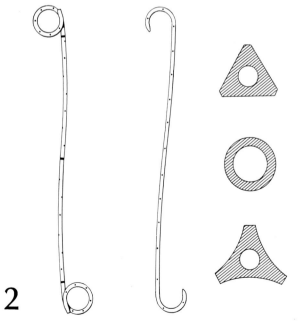

2

2 All ureteric stents are self-retaining due to their design. Polyurethane stents take the form of a pigtail, whereas silicone rubber stents are arranged in a JJ. Cross-sectional design of the stent, e.g. triangular or round, and the diameter of the lumen may influence urine flow, but this is largely influenced by the diameter of the stent chosen.

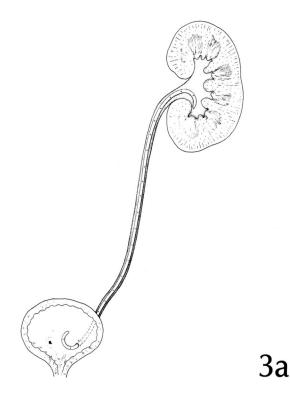

3a

3a–c The decision regarding the length of stent to be used is important. For most patients a stent length of 24–26 cm will suffice, and the correct length is estimated from the abdominal radiograph and confirmed during the operation by use of a ureteric catheter.

It is possible to insert ureteric stents without radiographic screening facilities, but an image intensifier is recommended for all cases of ureteric stent insertion unless the stent is inserted under direct vision through a ureteroscope, so that the precise position of the stent may be checked intraoperatively.

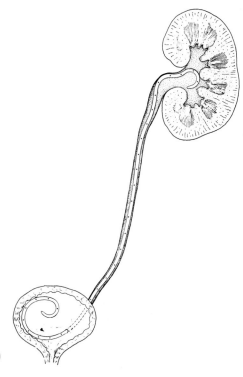

3b

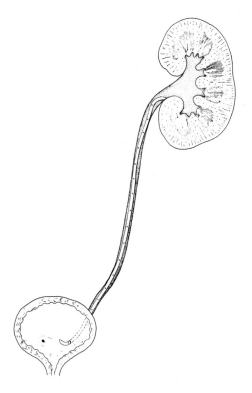

3c

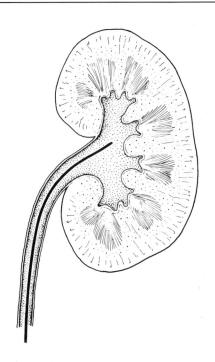

4

Operation

RETROGRADE STENT INSERTION

4 After identification of the ureteric orifice, ureteropyelography is carried out to clarify the ureteric and renal anatomy. The presence of contrast medium in the collecting system ensures the correct placement of the proximal end of the stent in the renal pelvis.

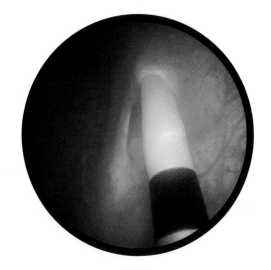

5

5 A soft-tipped 0.038 inch (0.96 mm) diameter guidewire is inserted through the instrument channel of the cystoscope until it just protrudes beyond the end of the Albarran bridge. The tip of the wire is introduced into the ureteric orifice by movement of the cystoscope, and the wire is advanced to the level of the renal pelvis. The position of the wire is checked by fluoroscopic screening. The ureteric stent is placed over the stiff end of the guidewire and advanced into the cystoscope. The pusher, a hollow plastic tube the same diameter as the stent, is also placed over the guidewire.

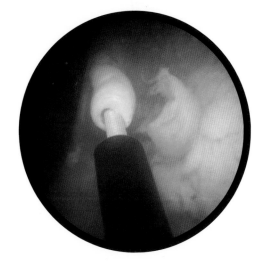

6

6 The stent is advanced into the ureteric orifice, while the stiff end of the guidewire is held by an assistant. The stent is advanced towards the renal pelvis using the pusher, its position being checked periodically by fluoroscopy.

7 Once the stent has passed into the pelvis, the pusher is firmly grasped and the guidewire is slowly withdrawn for approximately 5 cm. Fluoroscopic screening will confirm that the proximal part of the stent lies coiled within the renal pelvis, and the guidewire is withdrawn through the stent.

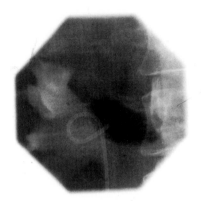

7

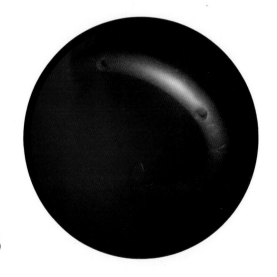

8

8 Once the guidewire reaches the junction between the stent and pusher, the distal tip of the stent will curl up into the bladder. There should be no more than 1–2 cm of stent protruding from the ureteric orifice.

Occasionally, it is necessary to reposition the distal end of the stent by grasping it with biopsy forceps and gently advancing the protruding portion of the stent into the ureter.

9 The position of the stent is checked by fluoroscopy, the bladder is emptied and the cystoscope sheath is removed.

Small stents (less than 4.8 Fr in diameter) can be inserted during ureteroscopy. The technique of insertion is exactly the same as that outlined above, but care must be taken to avoid inserting the stent too far up the ureter.

Ureteric stents may also be placed under local anaesthetic using a flexible cystoscope. The diameter of the working port of the flexible cystoscope (maximum 6 Fr) will limit the choice of size of stent to 4.7 or 4.8 Fr.

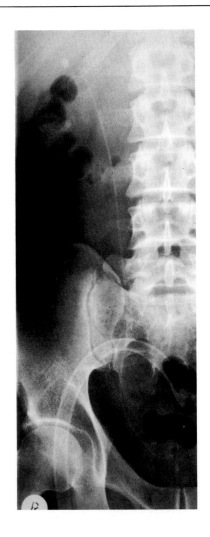

9

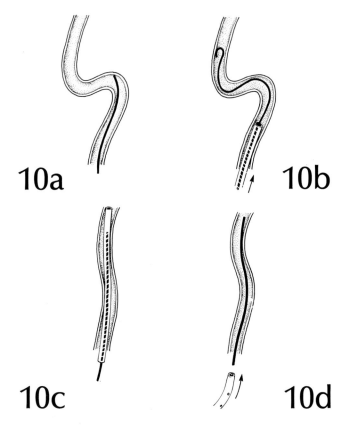

10a–d In certain instances, soft flexible stents will not pass a tortuous or tight ureteric narrowing, and it may be necessary to use a stiffer stent or guidewire. If this manoeuvre fails, the guidewire should be inserted up to the tortuosity and a stiff open-ended catheter inserted over the guidewire. The wire is then exchanged for a floppy-tipped J wire, which can be manoeuvred proximal to the tortuosity and into the renal pelvis. The catheter is then advanced beyond the tortuosity and the J wire is exchanged for a stiffer guidewire. The catheter is removed, and the stent is inserted over the stiffer wire.

ANTEGRADE STENT INSERTION

Antegrade insertion of ureteric stents is necessary if it proves impossible to gain access to the ureter from the bladder, if retrograde passage through a ureteric stricture is impossible, or during percutaneous endoscopic procedures. The antegrade approach influences the choice of stent. Unless the stent is inserted under direct vision during an endoscopic operation, it may have insufficient torque to enable it to pass antegradely through a narrow percutaneous track. Therefore, most stents inserted antegradely should be of polyethylene construction.

11 A soft-tipped flexible guidewire, a J wire or other floppy-tipped wire is inserted under fluoroscopic control through a percutaneous nephrostomy track that has been dilated to at least 10 Fr. The wire is manipulated through the ureteropelvic junction and advanced distally along the ureter and into the bladder. It may be necessary to dilate a narrowed segment of ureter with a balloon dilator before insertion of the stent, which is threaded over the guidewire together with the pusher; both pusher and stent are advanced over the guidewire and down the ureter under fluoroscopic control.

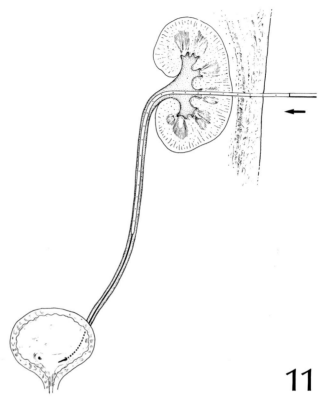

11

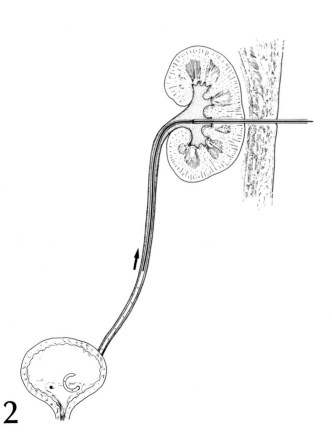

12

12 Once the stent appears to be lying in the bladder, the guidewire is withdrawn until the distal pigtail is seen on fluoroscopy to coil up within the bladder. The guidewire is then removed, and the proximal pigtail loop will coil up in the renal pelvis. The pusher is then removed from the track. A small nephrostomy tube may be left *in situ* for 24 h if desired to tamponade the track, but this is not always necessary.

STENT REMOVAL

13 Indwelling stents can be removed under local or general anaesthetic according to the patient's and surgeon's preferences. When local anaesthesia is used, lignocaine gel is inserted into the urethra 5 min before starting the procedure. A flexible or rigid cystoscope can be introduced and a grasping or biopsy forceps passed through the operating channel. The stent is then grasped with the forceps and withdrawn under vision.

If a stent with a magnetic tip has been used, an alternative method is simply to insert a magnetic remover into the bladder via the urethra under local anaesthesia, and once the tip of the remover makes contact with the magnetic tip of the stent, both remover and stent can be gently withdrawn through the urethra. This procedure sometimes fails, particularly if there is any encrustation on the stent, and the routine use of magnetic tip stents is not recommended.

Ureteric stents intended for short-term use, i.e. less than 1 week, can be supplied with a long nylon suture attached to the distal end. This suture is withdrawn through the urethra when the cystoscope sheath is removed after insertion, and it should be trimmed so that approximately 10 cm of nylon extend beyond the external urethral meatus. When the stent is due for removal, the nylon suture is simply pulled, and the stent is removed without the need for anaesthesia.

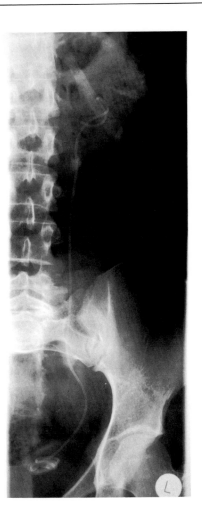

13

IMPORTANT - MEDICAL INFORMATION

Name: ....

If your ureteric stent has not been removed by:

Date: ....

Please contact the following Doctor:

Name: ....

Phone: ....

URETERIC STENTS

A small tube has been placed in the ureter to connect the kidney with the bladder as part of your treatment. This stent is not permanent and may block if it is left in for too long.

Sometimes there is pain, frequency of urination and slight bleeding in the urine. These symptoms usually settle down a few days after the operation. If they persist or if you experience pain in your side or feel hot and shivery, consult your Doctor.

This card was supplied as a service to Urology by:

LEWIS MEDICAL

14

Postoperative care

Antibiotic therapy is continued in high-risk patients, but the most important aspect of care is the maintenance of a stent register, in which details of all patients undergoing stent insertion are carefully recorded together with the dates of removal.

14 Instructions are given to each patient who has a stent inserted.

IMPORTANT
THIS PATIENT HAS A URETERIC STENT IN PLACE

Date Inserted ....   Date Removed ....

Stent Size .... fr/fg   Stent Length .... cms

Lewis Medical Ltd. 826 Green Lanes, London N21 2RT

Tel: 081-360 7273

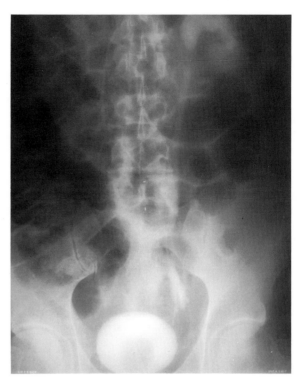

Complications

15 Perforation of the ureter may occur due to injudicious use of the guidewire. If this is recognized during the procedure, the guidewire should be removed and the stent reinserted correctly.

15

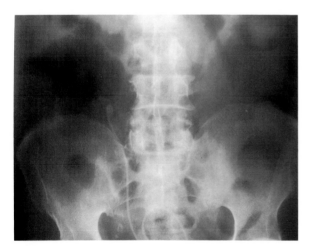

16

16 Occasionally, the stent is erroneously placed in the upper ureter and not in the pelvis. This happens when preinsertion ureterography is not performed, and therefore the ureteric anatomy is not adequately delineated. It may also occur if the procedure is not carried out under screening.

Extravasation of urine will occur if perforation of the ureter is not recognized at the time and may require percutaneous nephrostomy drainage.

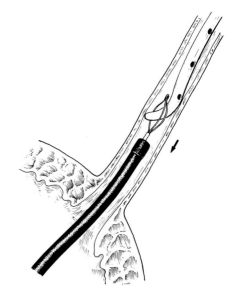

17 If the stent is inadvertently pushed up the ureter, it will be necessary to remove it by ureteroscopy and the use of a helical or flat wire basket.

17

Early postoperative complications are loin pain and haematuria due to trauma or irritation by the stent, infection secondary to the presence of foreign material in the urinary tract, and irritative symptoms of frequency and dysuria caused by trigonitis.

A long-term but important complication is the development of encrustation after 4 weeks, which may produce an increase in irritative symptoms and stent blockage. Although this can occur at an alarming rate in patients who form recurrent stones, this complication is entirely avoidable if individual stents are not left in place for more than 6 weeks. In extreme cases, extracorporeal shockwave lithotripsy may be required to disintegrate the encrustation before stent removal, and there are reports of encrustation being so great that endoscopic stent removal is impossible[4].

Extravasation of urine will occur if perforation of the ureter is not recognized at the time of stent insertion. This should be suspected if a patient complains of severe loin pain. The stent should be removed immediately, and if possible, reinserted. Preliminary percutaneous nephrostomy drainage may be required[5].

References

1. Zimskind PD, Fetter TR, Wilkerson JL. Clinical use of long term indwelling silicone rubber ureteral splints inserted cystoscopically. *J Urol* 1967; 97: 840–4.

2. Hepperlen TW, Mardis HK, Kammandel H. Self retained internal ureteral stents: a new approach. *J Urol* 1978; 119: 731–4.

3. Finney RP. Experience with new JJ ureteral catheter stent. *J Urol* 1978; 120: 678–81.

4. Pollard SG, MacFarlane R. Symptoms arising from JJ ureteral stents. *J Urol* 1988; 139: 37–8.

5. Saltzman B. Ureteral stents. Indications, variations and complications. *Urol Clin North Am* 1988; 15: 481–91.

Illustrations by Paul Richardson

Endoscopic treatment of ureteric strictures

Mohamed A. Ghoneim MD
Professor of Urology, Urology and Nephrology Centre, Mansoura, Egypt

Although the accepted treatment for urodynamically significant strictures of the ureter is by open surgical procedures, attention has recently been drawn to the potential for endourological manipulations.

Principles and justification

Indications

The endourological approach may be indicated in short strictures, particularly if they are of recent onset. Inflammatory strictures of bilharzial or tuberculous origin can often be successfully treated if they are in the formative stage before the development of excessive fibrosis in the ureteric wall and periureteric tissues. Again, endourological management offers an attractive alternative for the treatment of iatrogenic strictures that develop as a complication of surgery on the ureter or following ureterointestinal reimplantation. They may save the patient an open surgical revision, which is associated with a high incidence of complications.

Preoperative preparation

Urine culture, intravenous urography and a retrograde ureterogram are necessary. Radionuclide imaging and a diuretic renogram are performed to evaluate renal function and the response to diuresis. A preliminary percutaneous nephrostomy provides several advantages: it allows the performance of antegrade pyelography and/or a pressure–flow study; it reduces pyelotubular backflow during ureteroscopy; and it may be used as an access for antegrade dilatation of proximal strictures.

Operation

Principles

In general, the procedure involves three principles:

1. Visualization of the strictured segment by ureteroscopy. This is critical to allow threading of a guidewire through the lumen of the stenosed segment, the opening of which is often eccentric.
2. Dealing with the strictured segment by balloon dilatation or incision.
3. Intubation of the ureter for a period of 4 weeks using a JJ ureteric stent.

These procedures are carried out under general or spinal anaesthesia. The patient is placed in the lithotomy position if a retrograde approach is utilized, or in the prone position if an antegrade technique is required. An endoscopic table with a facility for fluoroscopy is mandatory.

Instrumentation

1a–c In addition to standard endoscopes, the following instruments are necessary to carry out these procedures: (1) A 7-Fr angioplasty balloon catheter (*Illustration 1a*), the length of the balloon being 4 cm. At an inflation pressure of 60 psi (4.4 kPa), the outside diameter is 6 mm. Inflation may be carried out manually or with the help of a mechanical device; (2) a right-angled diathermy electrode (*Illustration 1b*); and (3) a cold knife that slides on a guidewire for safety and stability (*Illustration 1c*).

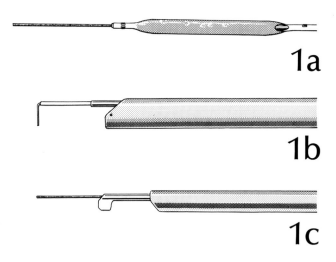

1a

1b

1c

Retrograde balloon dilatation of a ureteric stricture

2 Preliminary panendoscopy is carried out to inspect the urethra and the urinary bladder, and to identify the ureteric orifices. The intramural part of the affected ureter is dilated up to 7 Fr with a series of ordinary ureteric catheters. A 9.5-Fr semirigid ureteroscope is then advanced up the ureter until the pathological segment is reached. Under visual and fluoroscopic control, a guidewire (with a flexible tip, 0.89 mm (0.035 inches) diameter and 150 cm length) is threaded through the opening of the stricture.

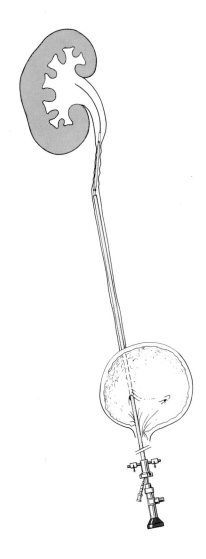

2

3   Once the guidewire has passed successfully an angioplasty balloon catheter is advanced over it through the central channel of the ureteroscope. With the help of the two radio-opaque markers on the balloon, its position is adjusted to the centre of the stenosed segment. The balloon is fully inflated by air or by contrast medium, and dilatation is maintained for 3–5 min. The efficiency of dilatation is tested by retrograde ureterography or by an antegrade study if a preliminary percutaneous nephrostomy has been performed. If the result is not satisfactory the procedure is repeated for a further 5 min and so on.

When an acceptable degree of dilatation is achieved the ureteroscope is advanced past the treated segment up the proximal ureter. The guidewire is adjusted to lie in the proximal collecting system. The ureteroscope is withdrawn and a JJ stent of a suitable length and of silicone material is advanced over the guidewire. Its final position is checked by fluoroscopy. The stent is removed 4–6 weeks later, and a check intravenous pyelogram is carried out. Significant decompression can be achieved with this procedure.

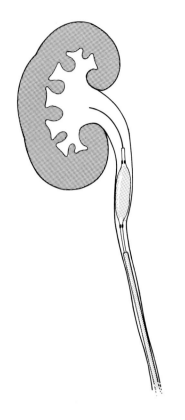

3

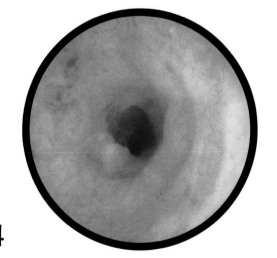

4

Endoscopic incision of a ureteric stricture with a diathermy needle electrode

4   Following preliminary panendoscopy, the intramural segment of the affected side must be dilated adequately to accommodate an operating ureteroscope (12.5 Fr). The ureteroscope is then advanced up the ureter until the affected segment is reached.

5 A flexible guidewire (0.94 mm (0.037 inches) diameter and 130 cm length) is threaded through the narrow segment.

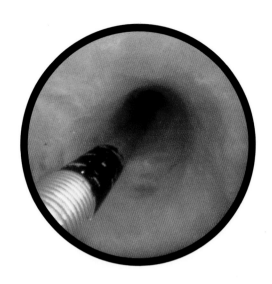

5

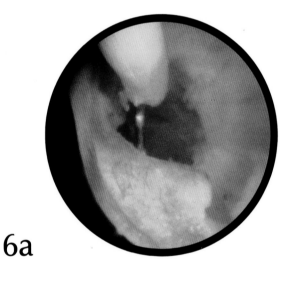

6a

6a, b The stricture is incised with a right-angled diathermy electrode. Careful small cuts are made in a posterolateral orientation until an adequate calibre of the lumen is achieved.

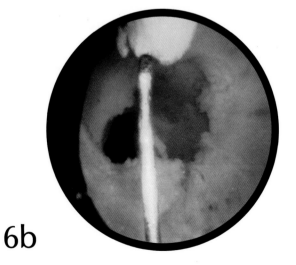

6b

7 The ureteroscope is advanced through the incised segment and up the proximal ureter. A second guidewire is introduced through the central channel of the instrument to reach the proximal collecting system, the ureteroscope is withdrawn, and a JJ stent is advanced over the guidewire.

The stent is removed 4–6 weeks later. A follow-up intravenous urogram is carried out and should demonstrate significant improvement in the configuration of the renal unit.

Endoscopic incision of a ureteric stricture with a cold knife

As an alternative, a ureteric stricture may be incised with a cold knife. The ureteroscope is advanced up the ureter to inspect the stricture as previously described. A guidewire is threaded through the stricture, and the knife is advanced through the stricture, guided and stabilized by the guidewire. The cuts are repeated until an adequate channel is established.

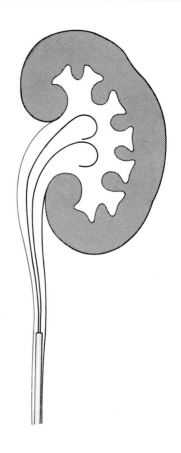

7

Antegrade balloon dilatation of a ureteric stricture

This approach is particularly indicated when dealing with iatrogenic strictures following surgery on the ureter or ureterointestinal reimplantations, when the retrograde approach is practically impossible.

8 A preliminary percutaneous nephrostomy is established preferably through a middle calix. The definitive procedure is carried out 48 h later to allow oedema in the stenosed segment to subside. A flexi-tip guidewire with a moveable core is introduced through the nephrostomy, and guided through the pelvis and down the ureter under fluoroscopic control.

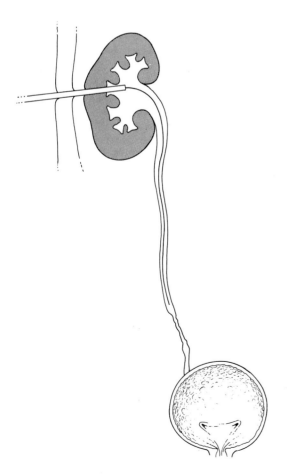

8

9 The tip of the guidewire is then softened by removing the core, and the guidewire is pushed through the stenosed segment. This can require repeated trials until successful passage is achieved.

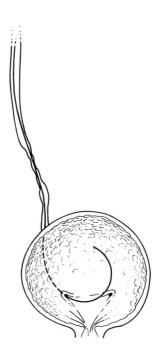

9

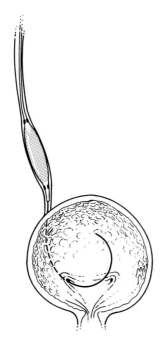

10

10 A balloon catheter is then advanced over the guidewire and its final position is checked by fluoroscopy aided by the two radio-opaque markers. Inflation of the balloon and dilatation are then carried out in the same manner as described for retrograde dilatation. Finally, the balloon is withdrawn and the guidewire is utilized for the placement of a JJ stent.

Comments

Endourological treatment of ureteric strictures is a useful approach in selected cases in which the pathology is not advanced. The stricture should be short in length and without extensive periureteric fibrosis. The approach is of particular value for strictures of iatrogenic aetiology, particularly those following ureterointestinal reimplantation. Difficult and complicated surgery may be avoided.

These procedures need further experience and refinement. The possibility of making an incision with a laser beam would permit the use of finer and more flexible instruments. The placement of internal stents made from hydrogels with improved biocompatibility also needs to be tried.

Illustrations by Peter Cox

Endoscopic correction of vesicoureteric reflux: the 'Sting'

B. O'Donnell MCh, FRCS, FRCSI, FAAP(Hon)
Professor of Paediatric Surgery, Royal College of Surgeons in Ireland and Consultant Paediatric Surgeon, Our Lady's Hospital for Sick Children, Dublin, Ireland

Principles and justification

1a, b Endoscopic correction of vesicoureteric reflux (the Sting) was first used in Dublin in 1984[1]. The principle is that at cystoscopy a small quantity of a paste containing polytetrafluoroethylene particles in glycerol (Polytef (USAN); Teflon, du Pont, Wilmington, Delaware, USA) is injected within or just under the orifice of the refluxing ureter at the ureterovesical junction. The bulge produced alters the shape of the ureteric orifice, preventing reflux without causing obstruction. Human application followed a successful experimental programme in piglets. The method of Subureteric Teflon Injection has become known as the 'Sting'.

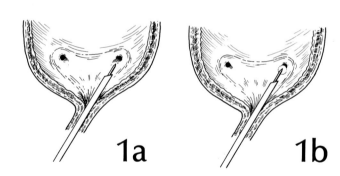

Indications

The procedure can be used to treat primary reflux of all grades and in all age groups[2]. The authors have also used it for neuropathic bladders and for persistent reflux following ureteric reimplantation. Paraureteric diverticulum is not a contraindication.

Contraindications

1. Combined reflux and obstruction: here the method may be useful but it is not definitive.

2. Very poor function in a kidney or segment of a duplex system: reflux is difficult to stop even with reimplantation and so nephrectomy or partial nephrectomy may be preferable options.
3. Punctured large ureterocoeles: where these give rise to severe reflux, endoscopic correction is difficult because of the poor backing bladder wall.
4. Severe granular cystitis is, as with contemplated ureteric reimplantation, a partial contraindication.
5. Two previous well-placed Stings.

Preoperative

Assessment

If the micturating cystogram shows severe degrees of reflux (grade IV or V out of five on the International Classification), then a radioisotope scan should be performed, using dimercaptosuccinic acid (DMSA), to assess the presence and extent of any scarring. Probably one-third of patients who come to intervention already have some scarring and this is particularly important as patients with scarred kidneys need to be followed for life.

Anaesthesia

The procedure is normally carried out on a day-case basis. General anaesthesia is required for children. The operation is painless and the authors do not warn parents about any specific immediate problems. Perhaps one in 50 patients will bleed from the needle hole but bleeding is always slight and has never required intervention.

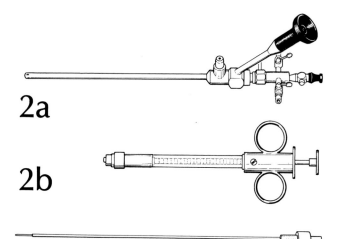

2a

2b

2c

Instruments

2a–c Endoscopes for this procedure have been made by Wolf (Mitcham, UK). The standard model (11 Fr) (no. 8625.31) has an offset eyepiece which takes a rigid needle (5 Fr) with a short 6–8-mm tip of 21 s.w.g. The paste is viscid and a 1-ml glass Luer–Lok syringe (Wolf) is used for the injection. The infant version (9 Fr), suggested by Dr Peter Frey of Basle, allows the procedure to be used in male infants.

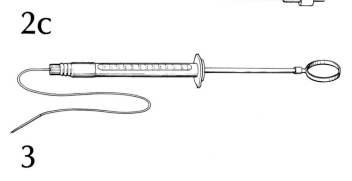

3

3 Alternatively, a standard 10-Fr (or upwards) cystoscope and a flexible disposable 4-Fr catheter designed by P. Puri and made by Storz (Tuttlingen, Germany) can be used.

The author prefers the rigid needle because it gives pinpoint accuracy and the position of the point of the needle can be altered more easily if this is required during the injection.

Operation

Position of patient

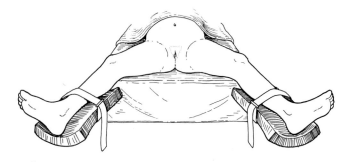

4

4 The patient is positioned on the table with the thighs extended and fully abducted. The purpose of this position is to flatten the base of the bladder and make the ureteric orifices more accessible for the needle. Orifices with severe reflux sometimes tend to be more lateral than normal.

Operative technique

A urine specimen is taken. The bladder is inspected and if there is severe granular cystitis it may be advisable to get this under control before proceeding. This sometimes necessitates 3–6 months' medication. The orifices are identified and are carefully inspected both from a distance and from close up. It is particularly useful if the existing submucosal tunnel of the ureter can be seen in the almost empty bladder. This gives the operator a better idea of the angle at which to insert the needle. It is important to keep the needle sharp as the mucosa tends to slip away from under the point before puncture. It is easier to put in the tip of the needle under the ureter when the bladder is almost full but, once it is in position, the effect of the paste is best seen with the bladder less than half full.

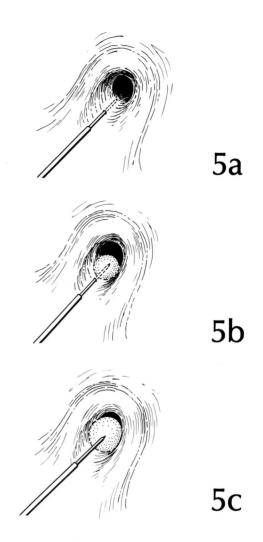

5a

5b

5c

5a–c The needle is inserted under the mucosa, about 2 mm distal to the ureterovesical junction, at *exactly* the 6 o'clock position, and it is then advanced *submucosally* about 5 mm in all. The needle should be visible under the mucosa. Injection is commenced slowly and the effect of each increment of paste is carefully watched. As little as 0.2 ml can produce a satisfactory result. Certainly 0.2 ml should be visible and should produce some alteration in the appearance of the ureteric orifice. If it does not, then the needle is probably too deep and the injection is being made into the bladder muscle. It is impossible to make the injection too superficial. Even if a white bolus appears just under the mucosa, no harm will come of it, and indeed this often produces the best result with the least paste. Injection is continued until the lumen is almost occluded and the roof of the ureteric orifice is stretched over the paste injection. The orifice of the ureter should appear either at the very top of the nipple or on the front. In a big orifice it may be useful to insert a ureteric catheter before the injection. In a really large orifice the endoscope may be put into the lumen, slowly withdrawn and the needle point made to spike or spear the mucosa just at the ureterovesical junction. The catheter is placed for the beginning of the procedure and then withdrawn towards the end.

The injection itself should be made by an assistant while the operator guides the needle and keeps it in exactly the right place. It is important that the injection should be made slowly and that the needle should be kept as still as possible, since enlarging the hole where the injection is carried out may allow paste to escape during or after the procedure.

A second injection may be made if the first does not produce the expected appearance. When moving to inject the second ureter, the operator may have to adjust position. When injecting the left ureteric orifice it may be necessary to step outside the right leg of the patient to get a good view. It is advisable when treating both orifices to inspect the first injection just after completing the second. Sometimes the glycerol in the injection will have been absorbed and what appeared to have been a satisfactory injection at the time appears less than complete. Inspection of the effect of the injection should always be made with the bladder almost empty. A full bladder may collapse a still incompetent ureteric orifice and give the operator the false impression that the injection was adequate. A second injection may be required at the time.

The maximum amount of paste used in any one injection has been 1.2 ml. This was in an exceptionally large orifice in a neuropathic bladder where the opening easily accommodated the instrument and the patient had massive ureters.

No attempt should be made to speed the injection and, rather than doing it more quickly, with experience the authors are doing it more slowly. There is certainly a learning curve and the best initial cases are girls between 4 years of age and puberty. It is advisable to do the cases in batches of two or three. This has the added advantage of conserving the paste.

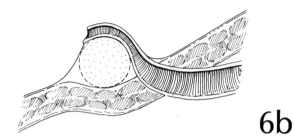

6a, b
The Teflon injection narrows the most distal part of the intramural ureter leading down to the ureteric orifice.

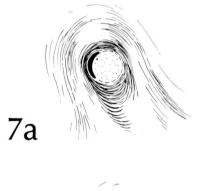

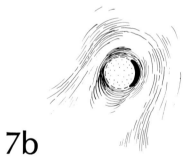

7a, b
If the appearance following injection shows that the hump is anywhere other than under the ureteric orifice the injection has been made in the wrong place, either too laterally or too medially.

Postoperative care

No specific warnings need be given to parents or patients. Although about one in 50 patients has passed some blood, there has been little in the way of painful micturition. Any paste left in the bladder quickly dissolves and is passed out with the urine. A micturating cystogram is essential 1–3 months after the procedure and 12 months later. In the past these patients have been followed for up to 5 years, but if the micturating cystogram at 1 year is normal the subsequent relapse rate is very small and no further cystograms are necessary.

Outcome

Present results are based on the concept that perhaps one in five Stings will have to be redone[3-5]. More than two injections in any one ureter are avoided if possible but the parents are told that a second injection may be necessary. In grades II and III (International Classification), the success rate after two injections is 95% or more. In grade IV, the success rate is 85% or more, while in grade V it is 75% or more. If two injections fail, an open reimplant may have to be carried out. The dissection of the ureter is not significantly more difficult in these cases and most of the extra 5 min spent is in preserving the bolus of Teflon for histology.

Reactions to Teflon

A number of Teflon granulomas — tiny seaweed-like excrescences at the site of the needle hole — have been seen. Many of these have been biopsied and show Teflon in the middle of the stalk. By ingenious experiments it has been shown that some small particles of the paste could migrate into other organs. The tissue reaction to these truly microscopic particles has been minimal. After 8 years' use in Dublin and an estimated number of more than 10 000 cases worldwide, there have been no reports of clinical reactions to migrated particles. Teflon is in wide commercial use and there have been no reports of ill effects to any of the thousands of factory workers engaged in its manufacture.

In response to the question 'Would you use this on a member of your family?', our answer would be an unqualified 'Yes'.

Substitutes for the Teflon paste are on trial and collagen appears promising. However, it is not satisfactory in the more severe grades of reflux and it has a documented tendency to disappear with time.

It is likely that endoscopic correction of vesicoureteric reflux using Teflon paste will increasingly become the method of choice for surgical intervention.

References

1. O'Donnell B, Puri P. Treatment of vesicoureteric reflux by endoscopic injection of Teflon. *B M J* 1984; 289: 7–9.

2. Puri P, O'Donnell B. Endoscopic correction of grades IV and V primary vesicoureteric reflux: six to 30 months follow up in 42 ureters. *J Pediatr Surg* 1987; 22: 1087–91.

3. O'Donnell B. Progress in the management of vesicoureteric reflux. *Postgrad Med J* 1990; 66: S44–S46.

4. Puri P. Endoscopic correction of primary vesicoureteric reflux by suburetic Teflon injection (STING): follow-up study in 123 patients. *Pediatr Surg Int* 1991; 6: 269–72. (Contains 73 references on the use of Teflon in urology and the experience of others with the Sting.)

5. O'Donnell B. Endoscopic correction of vesicoureteric reflux (the Sting): six years' experience. *Pediatr Surg Int* 1991; 6: 266–8.

Illustrations by Gillian Oliver

Catheterization

H. N. Whitfield MA, MChir, FRCS
Consultant Urologist, St Bartholomew's Hospital and St Mark's Hospital for Diseases of the Colon and Rectum, London, UK

Female catheterization is a procedure that is often safely delegated to nurses. Male catheterization is frequently performed by a junior doctor. It is in the male that there is a significant potential for causing trauma, which may have long-term sequelae, so it is important to understand the indications for catheterization and to appreciate the anatomy and possible pitfalls.

Indications

Patients may require an indwelling urethral catheter for any of the following reasons:

1. To relieve acute or chronic urinary retention.
2. To measure urine output.
3. Before surgery to reduce the possibility of inadvertent bladder injury, to increase the amount of room in the pelvis or to monitor urine output during and after surgery.
4. As part of the essential postoperative management of the patient, e.g. following transurethral resection of the prostate or urethrotomy.
5. To relieve intractable urinary incontinence.
6. Before certain investigations, e.g. urodynamics, cystography.
7. To obtain a urine sample for culture.

Preoperative

Prophylactic antibiotics are not necessary unless an untreated urinary infection is known to be present.

Operations

FEMALE CATHETERIZATION

The patient lies supine with her legs frogged. The labia majora are separated and the introitus cleaned with an aqueous antiseptic solution. The urethra is lubricated with local anaesthetic jelly. For most purposes an 18-Fr Foley catheter is suitable. The catheter is inserted for a distance of approximately 10 cm to ensure that the balloon lies within the bladder. When urine drains, the catheter balloon can be inflated safely.

Difficulty may be encountered if the external urethral meatus is stenosed. In patients with a cystocoele, the urethra may be positioned abnormally and the catheter will have to be directed posteriorly. In female patients with a hypospadiac anomaly, the meatus is located on the anterior vaginal wall and may be difficult to visualize, particularly if the hymen is present or if the vagina is stenosed. If the tip of the catheter is kept closely applied to the anterior vaginal wall, it is likely that the tip of the catheter will slide into the urethra.

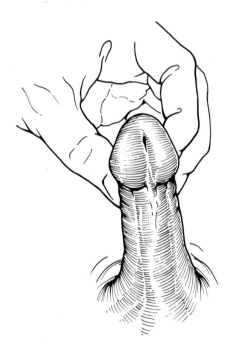

1

MALE CATHETERIZATION

1 To perform a male catheterization successfully the penis must be firmly gripped in a way that does not obstruct the urethra. The foreskin should be retracted. With the thumb on one side and the first and second fingers on the other side of the groove between the corpora cavernosa dorsally and the corpus spongiosum ventrally, immediately behind the corona, a firm grasp can be secured. After cleaning the glans with an aqueous antiseptic solution, 10–15 ml of a local anaesthetic jelly should be injected into the urethra and allowed to remain for 5 min. An 18-Fr Foley catheter can then be inserted.

2 The tip of the catheter will follow the 90° curve of the bulbar urethra if gentle pressure is exerted. At the membranous urethra there is the potential for the striated circular external urethral sphincter to be contracted and to cause a degree of obstruction. By asking the patient to take a deep breath and then to breathe out slowly and deeply, this muscle can be made to relax and the tip of the catheter can be passed further on into the bladder. Only when the catheter has been fully inserted into the urethra should the balloon be blown up.

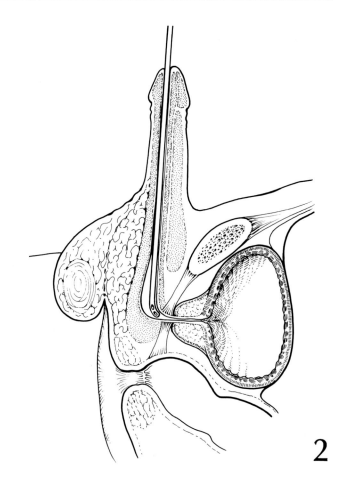

2

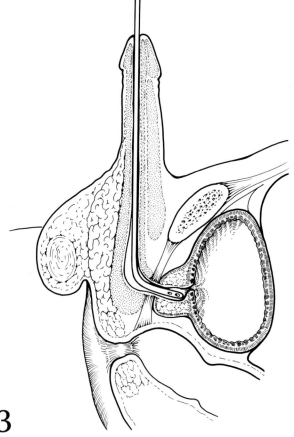

3

3 Difficulties can be encountered if a urethral stricture is present. In any patient who has had a prostatectomy there may be a shelf at the bladder neck and this can cause obstruction to the passage of a urethral catheter. In both circumstances a suprapubic cystostomy should be inserted. No attempt should be made to dilate the urethra or to use wire catheter introducers, except by an experienced urologist.

Postoperative care

Patients should be encouraged to maintain a high fluid input. The catheter, particularly where it emerges from the external urethral meatus, should be kept clean using normal saline. Discomfort at the meatus can be alleviated by applying local anaesthetic jelly.

Prophylactic antibiotics are contraindicated. It is inevitable that organisms would become resistant to any antibiotic given. Only if a patient develops a fever in the presence of a urinary infection are antibiotics indicated.

The frequency with which long-term indwelling catheters should be changed varies. Some patients block their catheters very quickly with phosphatic debris and catheter changes may need to be as frequently as 2-weekly. On other occasions catheters can be left for up to 3 months. There is little evidence that silicone coating of catheters reduces the frequency of changing a catheter.

Complications

In both male and female patients urinary tract infection, catheter blockage and bladder stone formation can occur.

In men, significant urethral trauma can be produced if the catheter balloon is blown up while the balloon remains within the prostatic urethra. Severe bleeding is likely to occur. This complication can be avoided by careful attention to the technique outlined above.

In women with a neuropathic bladder in whom a catheter has been inserted to improve continence, bladder contractions may tend to force the balloon of the catheter down the urethra, thereby causing urethral dilatation to such an extent that no catheter, no matter what the size of the balloon, will remain in the urethra. This problem can be prevented to some extent by anticholinergic drugs. On other occasions a reduction urethroplasty may be necessary; alternatively, the bladder neck may be closed and a permanent suprapubic cystostomy inserted[1].

In men a long-term urethral catheter may erode the penile urethra progressively to produce a hypospadiac deformity. This can only be cured by an extensive urethroplasty operation and a suprapubic catheter may be a more appropriate alternative.

There is evidence that the urethra is particularly sensitive to ischaemic damage in the presence of a catheter in patients undergoing open cardiac surgery or those with an episode of prolonged low cardiac output, e.g. following septicaemia. The resulting stricture in the anterior urethra can be very tight and extensive and require a two-stage urethroplasty.

References

1. Blandy JP. Cystostomy. In: Whitfield HN, ed. *Rob and Smith's Operative Surgery. Genitourinary Surgery.* 5th edn. Vol. 1. pp. 329–33.

Bladder biopsy

H. N. Whitfield MA, MChir, FRCS
Consultant Urologist, St Bartholomew's Hospital and St Mark's Hospital for Diseases of the Colon and Rectum, London, UK

Principles and justification

Bladder biopsies may be required for the diagnosis of malignant and non-malignant conditions. Excision biopsy of bladder tumours is described in the chapter on pp. 109–112. Bladder biopsies may be diagnostic in carcinoma *in situ*, interstitial cystitis and in some infective pathologies such as bilharzia and tuberculosis.

Preoperative

Although tiny cup biopsy forceps are available for a flexible cystoscope which can be used under local anaesthesia, most bladder biopsies will require general or epidural anaesthesia, although the patient can be managed on a day-case basis.

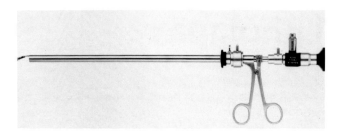

Operation

1 Rigid biopsy forceps are available which may be used through 20-Fr, 22-Fr and 25-Fr cystoscope sheaths.

The depth of the biopsy can be varied by changing the degree of bladder filling. With the bladder empty it is possible to include muscle in the biopsy. When the bladder is full a mucosal biopsy alone is obtained.

If random biopsy samples are to be taken then a minimum of three is required; these are usually taken from the right and left lateral walls and posteriorly. Flat areas of mucosal abnormality can be examined, with or without including muscle.

After the biopsy examination the site should be diathermied with a ball electrode to prevent any significant bleeding.

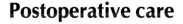

1

Postoperative care

A urethral catheter should not be necessary routinely. Prophylactic antibiotics are not indicated unless there is a pre-existing urinary tract infection.

Complications

Bleeding sufficiently severe to form clots can arise. The patient will then need to be catheterized and the clots evacuated. Urinary infection and septicaemia may occasionally occur.

Litholapaxy

H. N. Whitfield MA, MChir, FRCS
Consultant Urologist, St Bartholomew's Hospital and St Mark's Hospital for Diseases of the Colon and Rectum, London, UK

History

Evidence of bladder stone formation can be traced back to the Egyptian Empire of 3000–4000 BC. Over the centuries many horrifying but ingenious methods of removing bladder stones have been devised. In developing countries bladder stones, particularly in prepubertal boys, still occur frequently. However, in the Western world it is elderly patients with bladder outflow obstruction who most commonly develop bladder stones. Men and women with neuropathic bladder disorders, particularly in the presence of an indwelling urethral catheter, may also acquire bladder stones.

Principles and justification

When investigations reveal the presence of bladder stones it is almost always beneficial to the patient that these should be removed. Although open surgery may be required for the very largest, the majority are amenable to endoscopic treatment.

Preoperative

A prophylactic antibiotic should be given.

Operation

The instrument which is used will depend on the size of the stone. Although blind lithotrites are still available in many hospitals, the risk of causing damage with these is greater than with an instrument which is used under vision. For that reason either a stone punch, an optical lithotrite or an electrohydraulic disintegrator should be used.

It is often beneficial to dilate the male urethra so that the sheath of the operating instrument can be accommodated easily. A urethrotomy may provoke bleeding which obscures vision. It is also important, if bladder outflow obstruction exists in the form of prostatic enlargement, that the stone should be removed before transurethral prostatectomy, again so that vision is not obscured by bleeding from the prostatic fossa. Whatever instrument is used, the urethra should be lubricated liberally with local anaesthetic jelly.

Stone crushing forceps

1 Stones smaller than 0.5 cm in diameter can be crushed with forceps which can be passed through a cystoscope sheath.

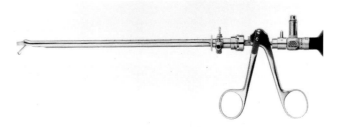
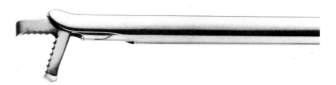

Stone punch

2 This instrument is passed into the bladder on its obturator. Stones of up to 1.5 cm in diameter can be grasped and crushed under vision.

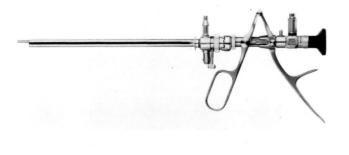

Optical lithotrite

3 The optical lithotrite is a large heavy instrument which must be passed with care when the blades are fully open. Stones of up to 3.5 cm in diameter can be grasped and crushed. When the stone has been crushed into fragments of 2 cm or less, the stone punch can be used.

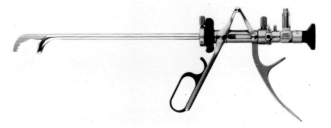
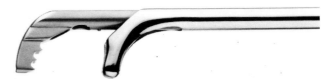

Electrohydraulic disintegration

Large stones must be disintegrated using an electro-hydraulic probe. A high tension spark is discharged across the end of the probe between the central core and circumferential electrodes. The strength and frequency of the impulses can be varied. Care must be taken not to discharge the probe when it is in contact with the bladder wall.

At the end of any procedure for crushing bladder stones all the fragments must be removed using an Ellick evacuator. Any coexisting bladder outflow obstruction must subsequently be treated.

Postoperative care

An indwelling urethral catheter is necessary, as much for the management of the bladder outflow obstruction as for the lithotripsy itself.

Complications

Trauma to the urethra can occur because the instruments used are large and cumbersome.

Damage to the bladder wall may arise if the bladder wall is included in the jaws of the instrument. This is a particular risk when the blind lithotrite is used. Electrohydraulic disintegration causes damage if the probe is discharged when lying against the bladder wall.

Extraperitoneal disruptions of the bladder may be treated by an indwelling catheter but intraperitoneal holes must be closed at laparotomy.

Bladder tumour resection

H. N. Whitfield MA, MChir, FRCS
Consultant Urologist, St Bartholomew's Hospital and St Mark's Hospital for Diseases of the Colon and Rectum, London, UK

Principles and justification

Indications

The resection of bladder tumours provides a very large part of the workload of a urologist. At the time of initial diagnosis, it is important that the tumour is resected so that a histological specimen is available. Recurrent bladder tumours found on follow-up cystoscopy may be suitable for cystodiathermy if the recurrence is small.

Operation

A preliminary cystoscopy should be performed to assess the size and site of the tumour(s). An Otis urethrotomy should be performed if the urethra is narrow to allow easy passage of a resectoscope.

The surgeon must make a preliminary assessment of whether the tumour can be resected completely. This is possible in those tumours that have not infiltrated more deeply than superficial muscle. The aim should be to resect the tumour level to the rest of the bladder wall.

With smaller tumours, it is often best to begin the resection towards the base of the tumour, particularly when a papillary growth has a relatively small stalk.

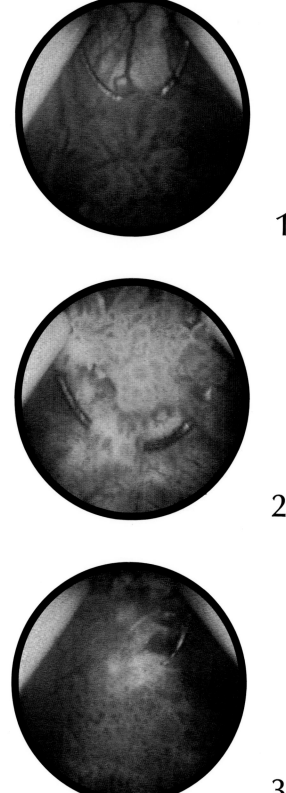

1–3 On other occasions when the tumour has a wide base, it is necessary to resect from the top or the side of the tumour downwards towards the base.

The degree of bladder filling will vary the intravesical anatomy very considerably. It is often helpful to have a continuous-flow Iglesias system, so that the position of the bladder tumour remains static. This is particularly important in tumours on the anterior bladder wall, which can tend to become inaccessible as the bladder fills.

Suprapubic pressure on a half-filled bladder may also help to bring the tumour into view. The fuller the bladder, the thinner the bladder wall, and the easier it is to perforate.

When tumours are situated on the lateral bladder wall, bladder filling may enable current spread to occur to the obturator nerves. This will provoke violent adductor spasm, which may itself provoke perforation of the bladder by the resectoscope. On such occasions, it is necessary to ask the anaesthetist to paralyse the patient completely to prevent this spasm.

4 Diathermy alone is sufficient for small areas of tumour, provided that adequate biopsies have been taken elsewhere.

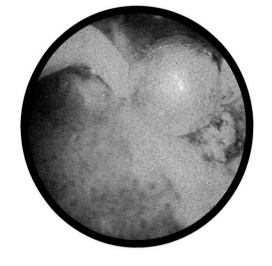

4

5 During the resection, bleeding points should be coagulated. When the resection is complete, the tumour base should be inspected and any bleeding points coagulated.

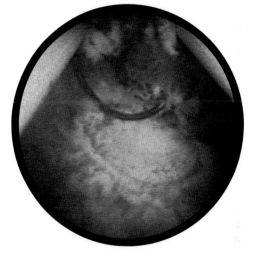

5

6 It is important to include muscle in the resection biopsy specimens, so that any invasion can be identified histologically. The resulting bladder defect must be inspected carefully for bleeding and for perforation.

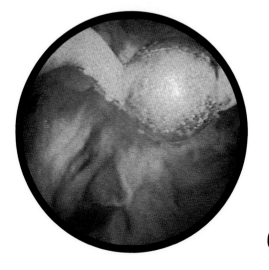

6

Postoperative care

Following the resection of a large bladder tumour, a three-way catheter with bladder irrigation may be necessary. On other occasions, adequate haemostasis can be secured, so that no catheter drainage is required.

Antifibrinolytic agents may have a role in the prevention of secondary haemorrhage following bladder tumour resection, in the same way as after transurethral prostatectomy.

Complications

Bladder perforation can occur. If the site of perforation is extraperitoneal, prolonged catheter drainage may be all that is required. Intraperitoneal perforation or the suspicion of it, however, necessitates a laparotomy, not only to enable the perforation to be closed but also to inspect intraperitoneal contents to ensure that there has been no diathermy injury.

Helmstein bladder distension

H. N. Whitfield MA, MChir, FRCS
Consultant Urologist, St Bartholomew's Hospital and St Mark's Hospital for Diseases of the Colon and Rectum, London, UK

History

A technique for hydrostatically dilating the bladder was first described by Helmstein in 1972. The value of this procedure in patients with infiltrating bladder carcinoma, for which it was first designed, has now been largely discounted[1, 2].

Indications

There are three groups of patients in whom the technique is worthwhile:

1. Patients, usually women, who have severe bladder instability and who have failed to respond to medical treatment.

2. Patients with very large papillary bladder tumours which, because of their size, make endoscopic resection impossible.

3. Patients who have intractable bleeding from the bladder mucosa, often after radiotherapy.

Preoperative

Because the pain from bladder overdistension is mediated through sympathetic nerves relaying between D10 and L2, high epidural anaesthesia is essential.

Operation

Specially designed Helmstein balloon catheters are available which have a capacity of up to 1 litre.

1 The catheter is inserted and the small balloon is blown up to retain the catheter within the bladder. The pressure balloon is then inflated under pressure with a pneumatic cuff around a 1-litre bag of saline. The dilatation balloon is inflated to a pressure equal to the patient's systolic blood pressure. A T connector enables intraballoon pressure to be monitored constantly.

The length and time for which the distension balloon remains inflated varies with the underlying pathology. Four successive 30-min periods have been recommended for patients with bladder instability[3]. For patients with large bladder tumours or with intractable bladder bleeding, a period of 6 h is recommended.

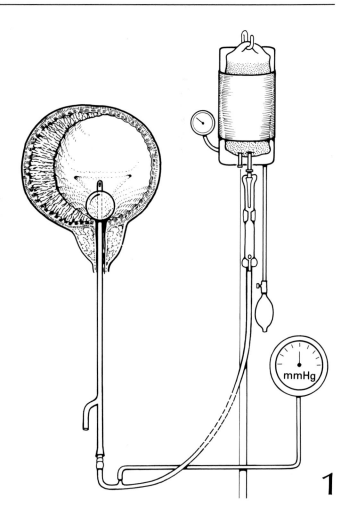

1

Postoperative care

A urethral catheter is required for 24 h. When the procedure has been performed for a large papillary carcinoma, the patient must be warned that particulate matter may be passed for a number of weeks.

Complications

Bladder rupture can occur during the procedure. For this reason the pressure of the distension balloon must be continuously monitored. Any sudden fall in pressure indicates bladder rupture and the procedure must be terminated. Although prolonged catheter drainage may be all that is necessary, formal closure of the bladder rupture is preferable.

The bladder may become atonic and require either prolonged catheter drainage or intermittent self-catheterization for a varying period of time.

Fragments of papillary tumour may cause urinary retention.

References

1. Helmstein K. Hydrostatic pressure therapy. A new approach to the treatment of carcinoma of the bladder. *Opuscula Medica (Stockh)* 1966; 9: 328–33.

2. Helmstein K. Treatment of bladder carcinoma by a hydrostatic pressure technique. *Br J Urol* 1972; 44: 434–50.

3. Dunn A, Smith JC, Ardran M. Prolonged bladder distension as a treatment of urgency and urge incontinence of urine. *Br J Urol* 1974; 46: 645–52.

Illustrations by Antoine Barnaud

Bladder transection

K. F. Parsons FRCS(Ed), FRCS
Consultant Urological Surgeon, Royal Liverpool University Hospital NHS Trust, and Director of Urological Studies, University of Liverpool, Liverpool, UK

Principles and justification

There have been many surgical procedures designed to reduce hypercontractility of the detrusor muscle of the bladder when it produces urinary incontinence. It has been held that the logical operation is to denervate the bladder, based on the assumption that the hypercontractility is neurologically mediated. This, however, is probably not the case, for in the majority of patients the cause of the hypercontractility or instability of the bladder is quite unknown, with no clinical evidence of neuropathy. Indeed this is borne out by the failure of the unstable bladder to respond predictably to a deliberate peripheral denervation or decentralization procedure. The operation of bladder transection is appropriate in these cases[1,2] and has the effect that the detrusor overactivity during bladder filling is reduced, and hence incontinence or nocturnal enuresis cured, while leaving the voiding phase of the micturition cycle unaffected.

The precise mechanism whereby the operation achieves its effect is still speculative but may relate to an alteration of modulating activity of interneuronal connections within the bladder wall together with the undoubted disruption of the myoelectrical conductivity of the detrusor syncytium[3].

There are two methods by which the bladder can be transected: either at open operation, or alternatively by the closed technique of endoscopic bladder transection. The closed operation requires considerable skill and experience in endoscopic urological techniques, and has probably entirely replaced the open operation[4]. Unlikely though it is that any attempt might be made to treat these patients other than by urological endoscopists, the original operation is described here, and it will be seen how closely it is mimicked by the closed technique.

Operations

OPEN BLADDER TRANSECTION

1 The bladder is exposed through a Pfannenstiel incision and opened by a transverse incision about 3 cm above the bladder neck. After coagulation or ligation of a few small arteries, the posterior wall of the bladder is picked up in the midline 2 cm above the interureteric bar, using two pairs of tissue forceps about 1 cm apart.

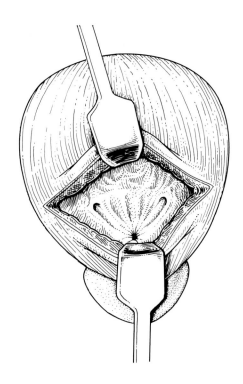

1

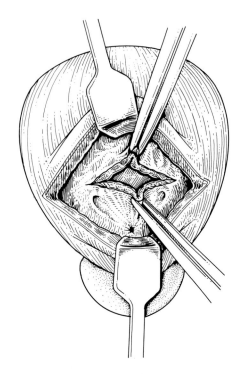

2

2 The bladder wall is divided between the forceps, opening the plane in front of the vagina or seminal vesicles. The posterior bladder wall is then incised transversely on each side to meet the lateral end of the anterior bladder incision, keeping well above the intramural ureter which can be identified with the aid of a probe if necessary.

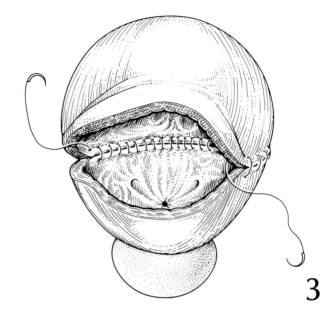

3

3, 4 The two parts of the bladder are sutured together with 2/0 chromic catgut. It is convenient to use two separate eyeless sutures, commencing in the midline posteriorly and working round each side until they meet anteriorly.

The wound is closed with drainage and a balloon catheter is left in the bladder for 7–8 days.

No attempt is made during this operation to divide any extravesical tissues, as some authors have recommended[5], since the results of both procedures are very similar, with a shift to the right of the cystometrogram and a significant symptomatic improvement rate of approximately 75–80%. Furthermore, the experimental evidence shows that no particular advantage would be expected by an extravesical neurotomy.

ENDOSCOPIC BLADDER TRANSECTION

The aim of endoscopic bladder transection is to mimic the open operation as closely as possible and to incise the full thickness of the bladder in a circumferential line which matches that of the bladder incision in the open procedure. As a preliminary step, after endoscopy of the lower urinary tract, each ureteric orifice is catheterized so that the course of the submucosal ureter can be readily seen, to allow the intravesical incision to be placed above it.

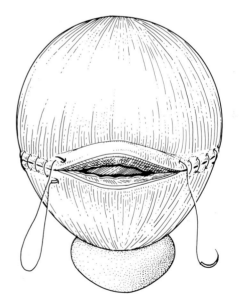

4

5 An irrigating resectoscope is essential for the operation so that the bladder volume can be set and held constant during the course of the operation by adjustment of the inflow and outflow valves. A Collings knife is used, and it is helpful to adjust the angle of the hot wire so that it will incise the mucosa at a right angle.

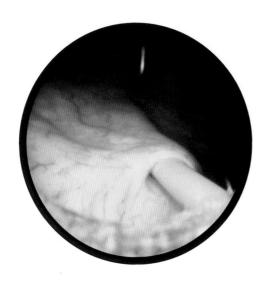

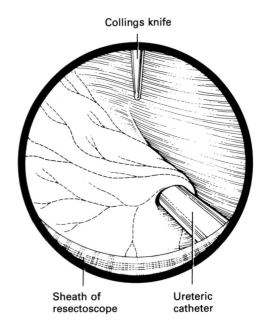

Collings knife

Sheath of resectoscope

Ureteric catheter

5

6 The proposed line of transection is then mapped using a series of small mucosal incisions which are positioned approximately 2 cm above the interureteric bar posteriorly, avoiding the intramural ureter on each side.

The line travels round each side of the bladder to the anterior surface where it lies some 2 cm proximal to the bladder neck.

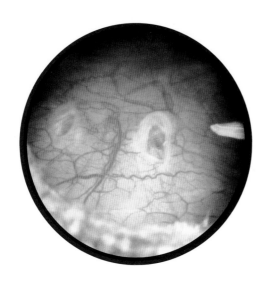

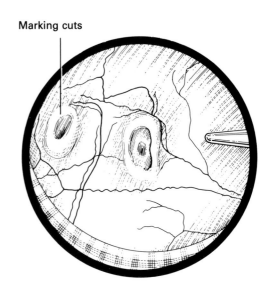

Marking cuts

6

7 The incision is then made, starting in the midline posteriorly, cutting through mucosa and muscle until extravesical fascia and fat are seen. As the mucosa is cut, so it will rapidly separate to reveal detrusor muscle fibres which themselves will separate.

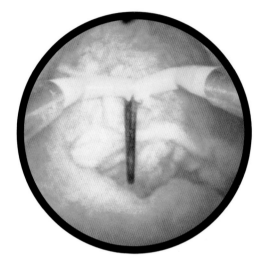

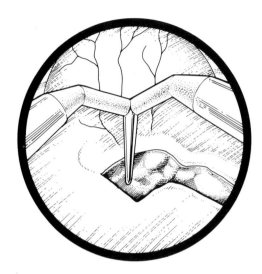

7

8 This process can be assisted by slightly increasing the bladder volume, but this should be avoided as the lateral incisions that are made for this will enhance the possibility of an 'obturator twitch', which is hazardous during this operation. The incision is completed round the side to the anterior midpoint.

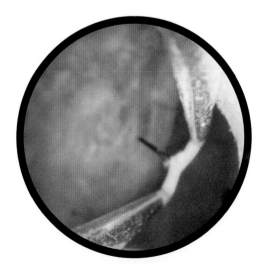

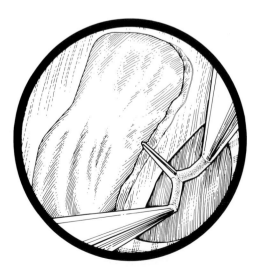

8

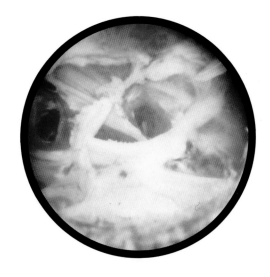

9   To complete the circumferential transection it is easier to return to the posterior midpoint and to cut across the back above the interureteric bar on the opposite side, extending the incision up the side to meet the contralateral incision at the front. Both marking and incising the front are facilitated by reducing the bladder volume.

When the initial incision is completed the cut can be widened by increasing the bladder volume, which allows remaining intact detrusor fibres to be dealt with individually. Often these will need to be lifted by the knife and can be surprisingly resilient.

Postoperative care

Haemorrhage is minimal, largely because the transection line is placed in the watershed between the superior and inferior vesical arteries. Any bleeding can be readily controlled by pinpoint coagulation diathermy. Extravasation is slight when great care is taken not to overdistend the bladder during the operation.

A 22-Fr catheter is used to drain the bladder for 8–10 days after the operation, during which period antibacterial therapy is administered.

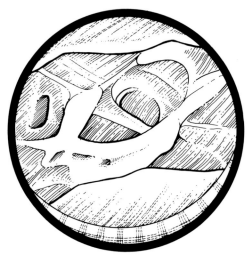

9

Outcome

Endoscopic bladder transection should replace the open operation with the expectation that the results will be identical. It should be limited to patients with urodynamically proven detrusor instability, often manifest as the enuretic syndrome.

Some 80% of patients have been shown to improve symptomatically, with a cure rate of 50%. In particular, bed wetting ceases. As with the open operation, improvement is not necessarily reflected urodynamically, nor can it be predicted by this investigation. A shift to the right of the filling cystometrogram is, however, a reasonably consistent finding. Morbidity is low and no patient has been worsened by the procedure. In those cases where the results are indifferent it is logical to repeat the procedure, and when unsuccessful, endoscopic bladder transection does not prevent a subsequent augmentation cystoplasty.

References

1. Essenhigh DM, Yeates WK. Transection of the bladder with particular reference to enuresis. *Br J Urol* 1973; 45: 299–305.

2. Gibbon NOK, Jameson RM, Heal MR, Abel BJ. Transection of the bladder for adult enuresis and allied conditions. *Br J Urol* 1973; 45: 306–9.

3. Staskin DR, Parsons KF, Levin RM, Wein AJ. Bladder transection – a functional, neurophysiological, neuropharmacological and neuroanatomical study. *Br J Urol* 1981; 53: 552–7.

4. Parsons KF, Machin DG, Woolfenden KA, Walmsley B, Abercrombie GF, Vinnicombe J. Endoscopic bladder transection. *Br J Urol* 1984; 56: 625–8.

5. Mundy AR. Long term results of bladder transection for urge incontinence. *Br J Urol* 1983; 55: 642–4.

Transtrigonal phenol

P. J. R. Shaw FRCS

Senior Lecturer and Honorary Consultant Urologist, Institute of Urology, London, and Consultant Urologist, St Peter's Hospital at The Middlesex Hospital, London and the Spinal Injuries Unit, Royal National Orthopaedic Hospital, Stanmore, Middlesex, UK

History

Denervation of the sacral nerves in order to reduce or stop bladder contraction has been used by a number of authors[1,2]. The technique of transtrigonal phenol injection of the pelvic plexus nerves was first described by Ewing *et al.* in 1982[3].

Principles and justification

Indications

Transtrigonal phenol injections of the pelvic plexus nerves are designed to reduce detrusor contractions in patients with detrusor instability or hyperreflexia and to diminish the symptoms of detrusor hypersensitivity in painful bladder conditions. This effect is thought to be due to a relative denervation which occurs because of the neurotoxic effect of phenol. The initial reports of the effect of phenol[3] have been affirmed by some authors[4,5], but not by others[6].

The experience reported by others enables the selection of a group of patients who will potentially derive short-term benefit from this technique.

In men there is a risk of impotence developing and therefore very few male patients have been treated. Good objective results are thus not available. It would be possible to use this treatment in men who are already impotent and who want a possible short-term relief of symptoms.

The dilemma arises as to how to treat the patient with severe symptoms of detrusor instability who does not respond to pharmacological manipulation, or where drug side-effects are too troublesome. About 50% of women over the age of 50 years who are suffering the effects of detrusor instability or hyperreflexia may expect to derive some short-term benefit and relief of symptoms. The effects of transtrigonal phenol do not generally last more than 9–12 months[6]. Patients with hypersensitive bladders or those younger patients with detrusor instability do not usually derive much benefit.

In those patients who seem to derive the least benefit, it may be worthwhile to repeat the technique to provide short-term benefit if the patient is keen to avoid major surgery, such as augmentation cystoplasty.

Preoperative

There is a likelihood that the occasional patient may develop detrusor acontractility after transtrigonal phenol injections. It is worth mentioning to the patient the possibility of postoperative retention of urine. Preoperative preparation is as for any cystoscopic procedure. The patient should be warned that a catheter may be left indwelling for 24 h after the procedure. Preoperative urinary tract infection should be treated, and all patients should have a single prophylactic antibiotic injection with the premedication or at induction of anaesthesia.

Anaesthesia

The patient is usually treated under general anaesthesia, though the procedure may be performed under spinal anaesthesia.

Operation

The patient is positioned in the lithotomy position. The technique is described as performed in the female.

The genital area, including the vagina, is cleaned with an antiseptic preparation. A preliminary cystoscopy should be performed to assess the bladder mucosal appearances and bladder capacity. Cystodistension for 5 min with an irrigant height of 100 cm and a measure of bladder capacity may precede the phenol injection.

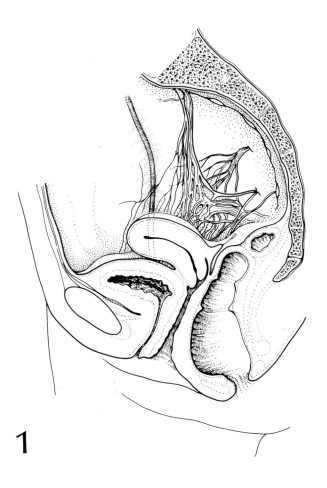

1

1 The aim of the procedure is to place 10 ml of 6% aqueous phenol in the region of the pelvic parasympathetic nerves.

A 23.5-Fr cystoscope with a deflecting mechanism is necessary for the procedure. A 30° telescope is used. A 45-cm long 20-gauge Shuttleworth needle is passed down the left catheterizing channel of the cystoscope for the left injection and down the right channel for the right injection. The needle is passed down the cystoscope until it comes into view in the bladder. It is not necessary to leave the stylet in the needle.

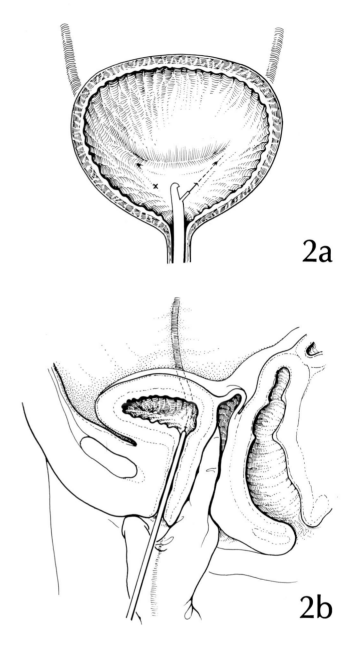

2a

2b

2a, b The needle should be inserted through the bladder mucosa midway between the bladder neck and the ureteric orifice. Once the mucosa has been penetrated by the needle, the deflecting lever should be turned to its full extent and the needle pushed through the bladder wall to lie behind the ureter. The line of the needle should be behind and along the course of the respective ureter. A finger should be inserted into the vagina to check the position of the needle. It is usual to feel the needle underneath the vaginal mucosa. If the needle has penetrated into the vagina, simply pull the needle out until the tip is seen in the bladder through the cystoscope and start again. The tip of the needle should be beyond the feel of the finger in the vagina.

The pelvic plexus nerves on each side are injected with 10 ml of 6% aqueous phenol. Each 10 ml of the fluid should be held in separate 10-ml plastic syringes. Care must be taken when injecting to avoid the risk of squirting phenol in the eyes or face. The surgeon should not look down the cystoscope while injecting. It is worthwhile to stop injecting to check visually that the injection is correctly placed. The use of a teaching aid or television camera helps in this technique, as the injection may be monitored without risk to the eyes. If resistance to the injection develops, the needle should be repositioned.

With a finger in the vagina, and an assistant holding the cystoscope, the bleb produced by the injection is usually palpable in the vaginal fornix on bimanual examination. The presence of a cold swelling developing just underneath the vaginal wall is usual. Provided the injection occurs without resistance and the swelling is underneath the vaginal wall, there is no cause for concern. If there is a swelling in the vagina at the end of the procedure, it should be massaged with a finger in the vagina to dispel it. If difficulty with the injection of 10 ml phenol is experienced, 5 ml will suffice. The procedure should be repeated on the opposite side.

When the needle is first placed, it may be too superficial and lie under the mucosa of the bladder, within the bladder wall behind the ureter, or within the ureter. There is no doubt that there is a learning process with this technique. If the needle is in the wrong place,

it should be repositioned. If there is doubt about the needle position, a very small quantity of saline should be injected through the needle and observed through the cystoscope. If a bleb is raised under the mucosa of the bladder, the needle is in the wrong place. When completed, the phenol injection should not be visible in the bladder. At the end of the procedure, a small amount of oozing from the puncture sites should be expected. A small-bore Foley catheter should be placed for 12–24 h.

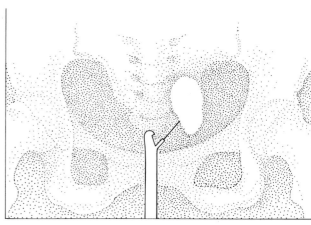

3 If radiological contrast is added to the phenol, the area of spread of the injection should be about 3 × 2 cm.

3

Postoperative care

The indwelling catheter should be removed the day after operation. Occasionally, patients develop retention of urine, and intermittent catheterization should be commenced. Only one of 94 patients developed a permanent acontractile bladder in the series of Rosenbaum *et al.*[6]

Complications

Care should be taken during the operative procedure to avoid injecting phenol into the area between the bladder and vagina. Vesicovaginal and ureterovaginal fistulae have been reported[5], but these are avoidable. Subtrigonal phenol injections should not be performed for this reason.

References

1. Ingelman-Sundberg A. Partial denervation of the bladder. A new operation for treatment of urge incontinence and similar conditions in women. *Acta Obstet Gynecol Scand* 1959; 38: 487–502.

2. Torrens MJ, Griffith HB. The control of the uninhibited bladder by selective sacral neurectomy. *Br J Urol* 1974; 46: 639–44.

3. Ewing R, Bultitude MI, Shuttleworth KED. Subtrigonal phenol injection for urge incontinence secondary to detrusor instability in females. *Br J Urol* 1982; 54: 689–92.

4. Blackford HN, Murray K, Stephenson TP, Mundy AR. Results of transvesical infiltration of the pelvic plexuses with phenol in 116 patients. *Br J Urol* 1984; 56: 647–9.

5. Cameron-Strange A, Millard RJ. Management of refractory detrusor instability by transvesical phenol injection. *Br J Urol* 1988; 62: 323–5.

6. Rosenbaum TP, Shaw PJR, Worth PHL. Trans-trigonal phenol failed the test of time. *Br J Urol* 1990; 66: 164–9.

Bladder neck Teflon injections

R. C. L. Feneley MA, MChir, FRCS
Consultant Urologist, Southmead Hospital, Bristol and Senior Clinical Lecturer, University of Bristol, UK

History

The concept of injection therapy for women with urinary stress incontinence was proposed in 1938 by Murless[1] who injected sodium morrhuate into the anterior vaginal wall. In 1973 Berg[2] injected polytetra-fluoroethylene (Polytef (USAN); Teflon, du Pont, Wilmington, Delaware, USA) periurethrally into three women whose urinary incontinence had failed to respond to conventional operative treatment, describing the procedure as 'Polytef augmentation urethroplasty'. Politano[3] promoted the technique and in 1982 reported a 70% success rate in the treatment of men and women. Few reports have substantiated his results, particularly in postprostatectomy incontinence. In 1983 Schulman et al.[4] treated women with stress incontinence by this technique, claiming a cure rate of 70%, but again few reports have repeated these results[5,6].

Teflon paste is a suspension of polytetrafluoroethylene particles in glycerine and polysorbate and is marketed in the UK as Ethicon Polytef Paste for Injection (Ethicon, Edinburgh, UK). The particles promote a fibroblastic reaction and increase urethral resistance. Schulman et al.[4] showed an increase in the functional urethral length and a decrease of 5 ml/s in the urine flow rate. Migration of the particles has been described but no serious morbidity has been reported.

Principles and justification

Indications

The main indication for periurethral Teflon injection (PTI) is genuine stress incontinence in women that has failed to respond to conventional techniques. The technique is simple and neither age nor obesity are contraindications to treatment. The method is not recommended for primary treatment; associated genital prolapse, bladder neck descent or cystocoele should be corrected by appropriate surgery. Detrusor instability is considered a contraindication but PTI has been used successfully in some patients with neuropathic bladder disorders associated with hyper-reflexic detrusors[7]. The injection may be repeated and the particulate deposits do not compromise subsequent surgery.

Preoperative

Careful selection is essential for patients with urinary incontinence to ensure that the indications are correct. A midstream specimen of urine should be examined by microscopy and culture and appropriate antibiotic therapy should be started if a urinary infection is identified. Urodynamic assessment should be performed to confirm the diagnosis of genuine stress incontinence and to exclude detrusor instability.

The patient should be warned of possible voiding difficulty requiring intermittent catheterization for a few days after the injection therapy which can be accompanied by burning discomfort in the urethra.

Operation

The procedure is normally carried out under general anaesthesia and is of short duration. The patient is placed in the lithotomy position, the skin is prepared and the region is draped as for a routine endoscopic operation. Urethroscopy and cystoscopy are undertaken initially to exclude local disease.

Two operative approaches have been described, involving either a perineal or a transurethral injection. The perineal injection requires a relatively wide-bore needle because the paste is a thick viscous material that is difficult to inject by hand with a syringe. This method has been superseded with the availability of equipment for transurethral injection, which is now the recommended route.

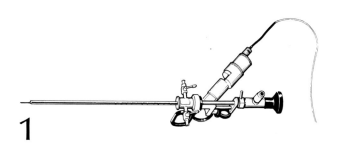

1

1 A dedicated endoscope with a cylinder and plunger is available (Richard Wolf, Mitcham, UK); 5 ml Teflon paste is introduced into the cylinder and the plunger is powered by a carbon dioxide gas cylinder that is activated from a foot pedal.

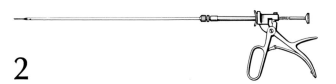

2

2 Alternatively there is a specially designed high pressure syringe, handle and flexible plastic tubing fitted with an end needle (Karl Storz, Tuttlingen, Germany) that can be passed through a 23.5-Fr cystoscope sheath and directed by an Albarran lever.

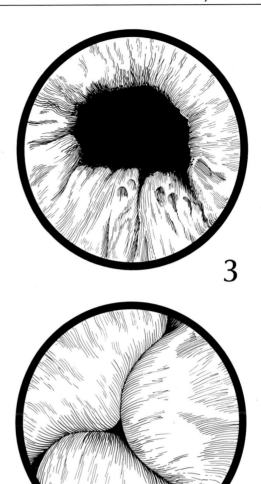

3 The bladder neck is visualized through a 5° or 0° telescope; the endoscope is then withdrawn so that the injection needle can be passed into the wall of the urethra about 1 cm below the bladder neck.

4 The initial injections of Teflon are normally given at 3, 6, and 9 o'clock until the lumen of the urethra is closed.

If subsequent injections are required, they can be introduced at other points at that level to facilitate urethral closure. The Teflon paste should not be injected too superficially into the submucosal layer of the urethra, otherwise it can be extruded as the needle is withdrawn.

Postoperative care

Continuous or intermittent catheterization 4–6-hourly may be required during the first 24–48 h after the operation; care should be taken to avoid overdistension of the bladder during this period. Pyrexia may be recorded in about 10% of cases; prophylactic broad-spectrum antibiotic cover is recommended during the first 2 weeks after the procedure.

The patient can usually be discharged from hospital 48–72 h after the injection. Dysuria is commonly experienced in the first week.

References

1. Murless BC. The injection treatment of stress incontinence. *J Obstet Gynaecol Br Emp* 1938; 45: 67–73.

2. Berg S. Polytef augmentation urethroplasty. Correction of surgically incurable urinary incontinence by injection technique. *Arch Surg* 1973; 107: 379–81.

3. Politano VA. Periurethral polytetrafluoroethylene injection for urinary incontinence. *J Urol* 1982; 127: 439–42.

4. Schulman CC, Simon J, Wespes E, Germeau F. Endoscopic injection of Teflon for female urinary incontinence. *Eur Urol* 1983; 9: 246–7.

5. Lim KB, Ball AJ, Feneley RCL. Periurethral Teflon injection: a simple treatment for urinary incontinence. *Br J Urol* 1983; 55: 208–10.

6. Osther PJ, Rohl H. Female urinary stress incontinence treated with Teflon injections. *Acta Obstet Gynecol Scand* 1987; 66: 333–5.

7. Lewis RI, Lockhart JL, Politano VA. Periurethral polytetrafluoroethylene injections in incontinent female subjects with neurogenic bladder disease. *J Urol* 1984; 131: 459–62.

Bladder neck incision

Patrick O'Boyle ChM, FRCS
Consultant Urologist, Musgrove Park Hospital, Taunton, Somerset, UK

History

From the early 19th century a variety of ingenious instruments has been devised to disrupt the prostate forcibly and permit catheterization. In 1834 Guthrie concluded that incision of the 'bar formed at the bladder neck' by a spring-loaded knife attached to a urethral sound was a precise and safe method of relieving obstruction. Bottini in 1876 introduced the Galvano cautery water-cooled 'incisore prostatico' and thus paved the way for the development of endoscopic surgery as we know it today. The enthusiasm of the succeeding generations of surgeons to exploit technological advances and completely remove obstructing adenoma has now been tempered by the realization that in some circumstances obstruction may be relieved by the lesser operation of bladder neck incision. Edwards et al.[1] emphasized that the procedure is easy to teach and learn and may be the operation of choice for the small benign prostate. Orandi[2] presented the results of a large series of bilateral bladder neck incisions now known as transurethral incision of prostate (TUIP), and showed that this treatment was effective in relieving obstruction produced by the small prostate and carries a lower incidence of complications than a full transurethral prostatectomy (TURP).

Principles and justification

Bladder neck incision is an attractive proposition due to the short operating time, short inpatient stay, short convalescence time and low incidence of complications.

Indications

The indications for bladder neck incision include bladder neck obstruction (including the dyssynergic variety), bladder neck stenosis and the management of the small prostate.

The classic indication is to treat the developmental abnormality which results in bladder neck elevation and fibrosis. Clinically this is manifest as the 'non-competitive stream' in childhood with symptoms rapidly deteriorating in middle age due to the development of early adenoma, resulting in the 'trapped prostate'. These cases are infrequent but visually dramatic as the bladder neck opens widely, and is most gratifying for the patient who subsequently voids with a normal flow for the first time in his life. Dyssynergic bladder neck obstruction, a poorly understood neuromuscular imbalance, is confirmed by synchronous pressure flow urodynamics. The treatment of choice is a single full bladder neck incision[3].

Bladder neck stenosis usually occurs after resection of the small prostate. The stenosis may open widely after incision, but may require multiple separate cuts with resection of the intervening fibrous tissue, or bladder neck resection to achieve a satisfactory appearance.

It is surprising how often a very small prostate produces a disproportionate degree of bladder dysfunction, with the development of chronic retention and an atonic bladder. The temptation to resect the prostate completely should be resisted. The bladder neck which is probably responsible for the obstruction will not be treated adequately by resection. Bladder neck incision will usually give a more satisfactory result.

Preoperative

The same principles apply as in the chapter on 'Transurethral prostatectomy', pp. 137–144. In addition to the equipment mentioned on page 138, a Collings knife electrode is used to introduce the resectoscope.

Operation

The objective is to produce a single clean incision in the 7 o'clock position, from just below the right ureteric orifice to alongside the verumontanum, completely dividing all bladder neck fibres in the line of the incision through to the outer part of the capsule. The microvideo operating system is particularly useful for this operation due to the magnified image on the video monitor which encourages very gentle strokes of the electrode as the bladder neck fibres pull apart.

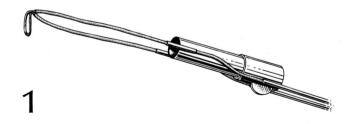

1

1 After endoscopic examination of the bladder and urethra the resectoscope is introduced with the Collings knife electrode. The ureteric orifices are carefully identified with particular attention to the distances from the bladder neck.

2 The position of the verumontanum is noted together with the topography of any prostatic adenoma which may influence the line of the resection. The bladder neck has the appearance of a wall of tissue preventing direct inspection of the bladder base.

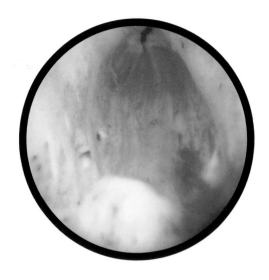

2

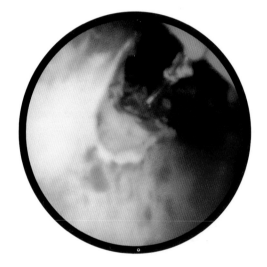

3

3 The incision is started cautiously in the 7 o'clock position, just inside the internal urinary meatus, dividing the mucosa and exposing the bladder neck fibres.

4 As the incision is deepened the bladder neck fibres can be seen to spring apart revealing further layers. They are progressively divided at this level by delicate diathermy incision until the capsule is reached.

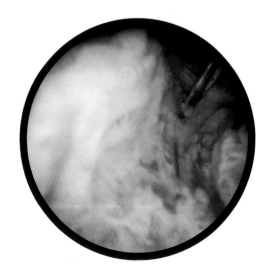

4

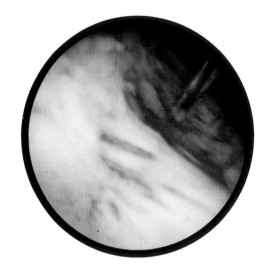

5

5 This may be recognized by the sudden transition of a glistening translucent cobweb appearance to accompanying small globules of fat.

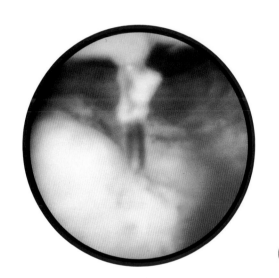

6

6 The incision is finally extended proximally to just below the right ureteric orifice and distally to alongside the verumontanum.

It should now be possible to view the base of the bladder with the telescope at the level of the verumontanum.

The line of the incision is inspected for bleeding vessels which should be carefully sealed with pinpoint diathermy. If mucosal bleeding is troublesome this may be conveniently dealt with by roller ball coagulation.

Finally, an 18-Fr three-way irrigation catheter is carefully inserted with the Maryfield introducer.

Postoperative care

The patient should be monitored exactly as for transurethral prostatectomy (page 144). Significant postoperative bleeding can occur, particularly when the incision is associated with small adenomas in younger men. Despite the short operating time this should not be regarded casually as minor surgery. Bleeding will invariably respond to light catheter traction, but particular care should be taken to avoid a blocked catheter and bladder overdistension, which may further disrupt the capsule and result in extravasation. Complications otherwise are minimal. The catheter is removed on the day after the operation following a single dose of an intravenous antibiotic (usually gentamicin, 80 mg) and the patient is discharged when voiding is satisfactory. A follow-up appointment with urinary flow rate measurement is carried out at 4 weeks.

References

1. Edwards LE, Bucknall TE, Pittam MR *et al*. Transurethral resection of the prostate and bladder neck incision: a review of 700 cases. *Br J Urol* 1985; 57: 168–71.

2. Orandi A. Re-operation after transurethral incision of the prostate (TUIP): 18 year follow-up. *J Urol* 1988; 139: 272A.

3. Turner-Warwick RT. The evaluation of urodynamic function. *Urol Clin North Am* 1979; 6: 51.

Prostate biopsy

Leonard G. Gomella MD
Assistant Professor, Department of Urology, Jefferson Medical College, Thomas Jefferson University, Philadelphia, Pennsylvania, USA

S. Grant Mulholland MD
The Nathan Lewis Hatfield Professor and Chairman, Department of Urology, Jefferson Medical College, Thomas Jefferson University, Philadelphia, Pennsylvania, USA

History

Since palpable carcinoma of the prostate tends to arise in the posterior gland, the earliest attempts at biopsy relied on an open perineal approach. With further refinements in endoscopic techniques, transurethral biopsy was extensively utilized, and although there was good diagnostic accuracy in patients with large volume prostatic carcinoma, patients with early stage disease were often not properly diagnosed. Core needle and fine-needle aspiration biopsies (FNAB) of the prostate, often combined with ultrasonic guidance, have now become the most widely used methods to diagnose prostatic cancer.

Whether the diagnosis of prostatic carcinoma should be established by FNAB or core needle biopsy is unsettled. FNAB has been used most extensively in Europe and has recently become more popular in the USA. The advantages of FNAB are that it is relatively easy to perform, requires no anaesthesia, has a very low complication rate, and allows rapid pathological interpretation. The main disadvantage is that it requires a cytopathologist who is experienced in the interpretation of FNAB for its performance.

Principles and justification

Indications

Patients in whom the diagnosis of prostate cancer is being considered are the group most often considered for prostate biopsy. Findings that are suggestive of prostatic malignancy include nodularity, marked asymmetry, induration and fixation on digital rectal examination or elevation of the serum prostatic specific antigen (PSA) level in the face of a normal prostate examination. Biopsy may also be used to assess the efficacy of definitive radiation therapy in a patient with previously diagnosed prostate cancer.

Preoperative

Patients should be screened to exclude a bleeding diathesis and refrain from aspirin ingestion for 1 week before biopsy. If the transperineal approach is used, shaving is not necessary, but the skin should be prepared with a cleansing solution (e.g. povidone-iodine). For the transrectal biopsy, oral antibiotics (e.g. co-trimoxazole or a fluoroquinolone) are administered 30–60 min before the procedure and continued for 2–3 days. A cleansing enema is usually given just before the procedure.

Anaesthesia

Prostatic biopsy can be performed under general, regional or local anaesthesia. Due to advances in technique, however, biopsies are now often performed without anaesthesia. The use of intermediate-sized 18 gauge core biopsy needles, a spring-loaded, rapid fire biopsy gun and the transrectal approach allows patients to tolerate multiple biopsies easily without anaesthesia. If the transperineal approach is used, anaesthesia with 1% lignocaine is needed. FNAB of the prostate is most often performed transrectally without anaesthesia.

Operations

DIGITALLY-GUIDED CORE BIOPSY

Although the Vim–Silverman needle has been used for many years, the 18 gauge core biopsy needle, with or without a spring-loaded biopsy gun, is preferred by most operators at present.

The patient is typically positioned in the dorsal lithotomy position. Either the transrectal or the transperineal approach can be used; each approach has advantages and disadvantages. The transrectal approach permits more accurate needle placement into the lesion and does not require an anaesthetic, but is associated with a higher incidence of septic and bleeding complications. The transperineal approach is associated with fewer complications, but requires local anaesthesia and directing the needle into the lesion is more difficult than with the transrectal technique.

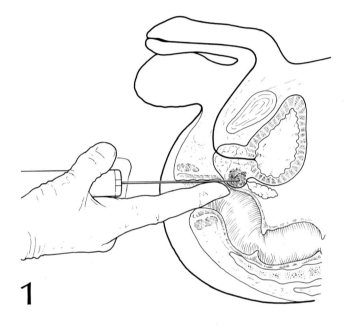

1 For the transrectal core biopsy, the biopsy needle is inserted along with the well-lubricated index finger. The lesion is palpated and the needle is advanced through the rectal wall into the lesion. If a biopsy gun is used, the needle tip is positioned at the lesion and the gun is activated, rapidly passing the cutting needle and then the outer sheath through the rectal wall into the lesion. The needle is removed and the core of prostatic tissue is recovered.

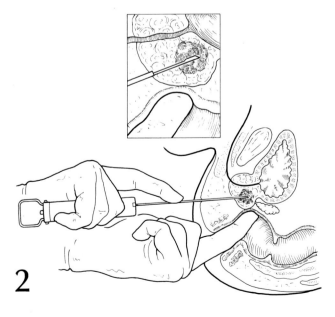

2 For the transperineal approach, the perineal skin above the rectum is anaesthetized with 1% lignocaine, and the deeper tissues and periprostatic area anaesthetized with a 22 gauge spinal needle. A small stab wound with a no. 11 blade eases the passage of the needle into the skin. The core biopsy needle is then inserted into the perineum while the examining finger is in the rectum. The needle is advanced under bimanual control to the suspicious area which is biopsied.

DIGITALLY-DIRECTED FNAB

FNAB of the prostate can be performed with the patient in the dorsal lithotomy, knee–chest position or leaning over the examining table with the feet spread apart slightly.

3 The Franzen (22 gauge) biopsy needle (Van-Tec, Indiana, USA) is prepared by aspirating approximately 1 ml of saline into the needle and expelling the saline.

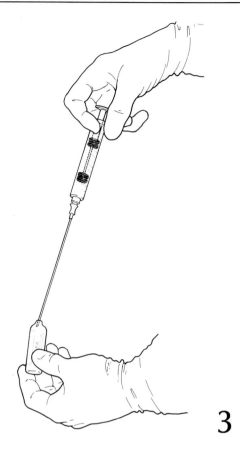

3

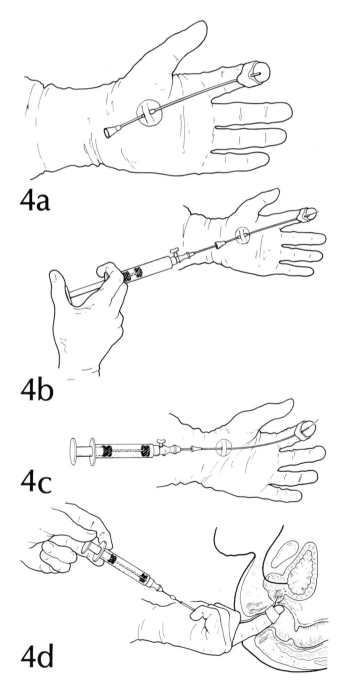

4a

4b

4c

4d

4a–d A needle guide is placed over a gloved index finger and a second glove may be placed over the needle guide. The index finger is lubricated, passed into the rectum and the prostatic abnormality palpated. The Franzen needle is then attached to a 10 ml aspirating syringe, passed through the glove into the needle guide and the needle tip is advanced into the suspicious area. Negative pressure is applied and the needle is passed using a back-and-forth motion throughout the area for 20–30 s. The negative pressure is released and the needle is withdrawn. Failure to release the negative pressure prior to removing the needle will result in faecal material contaminating the specimen.

Depending on the pathologist's requirements, the aspirate can be handled in one of two ways. Standard FNAB practice is to use an air-filled syringe to expel the needle contents onto a glass slide. A 'smear' is made by quickly passing a second clean slide over the drop expelled from the needle. The slide is then either air dried or placed in alcohol fixative for later staining.

Other laboratories now ask that the aspirate be drawn into a clean syringe using 2 ml of saline and then expelled into fixative solution.

The procedure should be repeated for a total of three or four collections. It is more comfortable for the patient if the examining finger is left in the rectum between collections.

ULTRASONICALLY-DIRECTED PROSTATE BIOPSY

Both core needle biopsy and FNAB can be performed under ultrasonic guidance. Core needle biopsy is more commonly performed in this way.

Whether transrectal ultrasonography (TRUS) is needed for all prostate biopsies is controversial. When a clearly palpable abnormality is present, the diagnostic accuracy of the digitally-directed biopsy *versus* that of the ultrasonically-directed biopsy appear similar in some studies, while other studies show improved accuracy when the biopsy is performed under ultrasonic guidance. Ultrasonography is very useful to guide prostatic biopsy when the gland is palpably normal but the PSA level is elevated, in cases where a suspicious gland has been biopsied previously without a definitive diagnosis or where the findings on rectal examination are subtle. Although prostate cancer is classically described as 'hypoechoic' on TRUS, it is now recognized that prostatic malignancies may also be hyperechoic, isoechoic or of mixed echogenicity. Since up to 40% of cancers may be isoechoic and therefore not well visualized on TRUS, random biopsies of 'normal' areas will increase the diagnostic accuracy.

The patient is prepared as for digitally-directed core biopsy and local anaesthesia is only used for the transperineal approach. The dorsal lithotomy position is most frequently used for the transperineal biopsy. Transrectal biopsy is usually performed in the lateral decubitus position.

Transducers are typically in the 5.0–7.5 MHz range and can produce real-time imaging of the gland. Newer biplanar probes allow scanning of the prostate in both longitudinal (sagittal) and transverse planes with the same instrument. The TRUS endorectal probe is prepared according to the manufacturers' specifications. All transducers are covered with a protective condom; some require that the condom be filled with 40–60 ml water as an acoustic interface. If the transducer requires a water interface, all air bubbles should be aspirated before insertion of the probe. The condom is well lubricated and inserted into the rectum. Transverse scanning is best for defining the lateral margins of the prostate and longitudinal scanning is most useful for prostate biopsy since the entire needle can be visualized and the exact tissue biopsied can be clearly identified. Biopsy can be performed 'freehand'; however, needle guides, either built into or attached onto the probe, are useful.

Transperineal ultrasonically-directed biopsy

5   The prostate is imaged by longitudinal scanning and the lesion is located. The core biopsy needle is placed in the needle guide and advanced into the previously anaesthetized perineum. The needle is then advanced into the lesion.

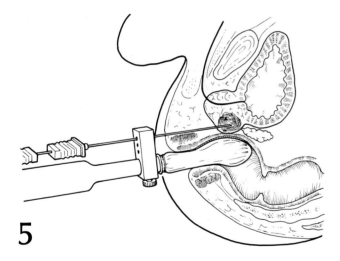

5

Transrectal ultrasonically-directed biopsy

6   The transrectal biopsy is usually painless, provided the needle does not pass through the anal sphincter. If the Biopty gun (C. R. Bard, Georgia, USA) is used, the needle is placed in line with the lesion and the gun fired so that the rectal mucosa and prostate lesion are rapidly penetrated.

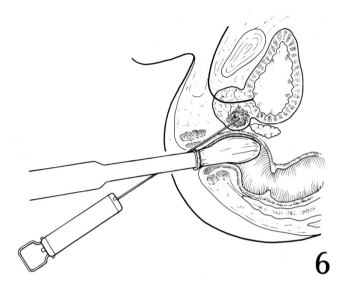

6

Postoperative care

Patients should be observed until they are able to void. Haematuria is common, but grossly bloody urine may require catheterization and irrigation. As mentioned previously, oral broad-spectrum antibiotics are continued for 2–3 days. Patients are asked to refrain from any heavy exertion for 1 week and should be informed that haematospermia is not an unusual finding several weeks after prostate biopsy.

Complications

Overall, transrectal core needle biopsy is associated with higher complication rates including haematuria (37%), bloody bowel movements (9%) and sepsis (2%). Complications of FNAB and transperineal biopsy are infrequent.

Further reading

Rifkin MD, Dahnert W, Kurtz AB. State of the art: endorectal sonography of the prostate gland. *AJR* 1990; 154: 691–700.

Rifkin MD, Alexander AA, Pisarchick J, Matteucci T. Palpable masses in the prostate: superior accuracy of US-guided biopsy compared with accuracy of digitally guided biopsy. *Radiology* 1991; 179: 41–2.

Illustrations by Paul Richardson

Transurethral prostatectomy

Patrick O'Boyle ChM, FRCS
Consultant Urologist, Musgrove Park Hospital, Taunton, Somerset, UK

Principles and justification

Transurethral prostatectomy is the most frequent operation performed by urologists. After the age of 40 years, every man produces a benign tumour of the prostate gland as part of the natural ageing process. Of these, 10% will require surgical removal for obstructive or irritative bladder symptoms and 95% of benign prostatic tumours may be safely dealt with transurethrally.

Patients and surgeons both owe an enormous debt to the persistence of the early pioneers of the transurethral approach in North America. In turn, outstanding developments in optical technology, in particular the Hopkins rod-lens system and fibreoptic lighting, have revolutionized endoscopic urology.

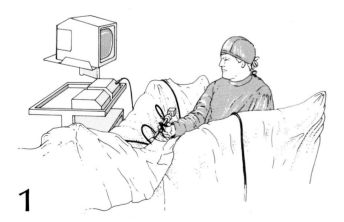

1 Additional refinements such as microvideo operating systems have contributed to the comfort and safety of the surgeon and facilitated the teaching of endoscopic surgery.

Indications

Transurethral prostatectomy is performed to relieve the symptoms of bladder outflow obstruction or to preserve renal function. Preoperative investigation should include urinary flow rate and ultrasonographic assessment of the bladder for residual urine, and of the kidneys for dilatation. This can conveniently be performed in an outpatient clinic by the urologist himself. Urography is not usually necessary.

Urodynamic evaluation may be helpful to detect detrusor instability, particularly in patients who have irritative bladder symptoms. This may not influence the choice of operation, but will forewarn the surgeon that it may take longer than usual for the patient to achieve postoperative control of micturition.

The size of the prostatic adenoma which may be safely removed transurethrally seems to attract much debate. In practice each surgeon will soon determine his personal limitation, which may well be dictated by the equipment and facilities available to him. The author has not been impressed by the results of resection of very large glands, which may be removed more rapidly and safely by open operation, nor by the concept of two or three 'staged' resections. The ultimate result for the patient depends not on how much tissue is removed, but on how much is left behind! Similarly, very small glands are notorious for producing bladder neck stenosis following resection. These are better dealt with by bladder neck incision or resection.

Preoperative

Many patients who require transurethral surgery are old, frail and have multisystem pathology. They require careful evaluation by both the surgeon and anaesthetist. An anaesthetic technique which reduces bleeding has obvious advantages for the surgeon, but the most suitable anaesthetic for the individual patient will be determined by the experience of the anaesthetist.

Significant electrolyte imbalance and anaemia should be corrected. A period of indwelling catheter drainage may be beneficial, particularly in patients who have chronic retention and a grossly overdistended bladder. A suprapubic catheter has the advantage of leaving the urethra and prostatic fossa unscathed and will provide a conduit for continuous flow irrigation which can reduce operating time. Urinary tract infection should be carefully assessed and treated before elective surgery. The author is convinced of the value of prophylactic antibiotics and favours gentamicin 80 mg intramuscularly at the induction of anaesthesia and on the morning of catheter removal. Compatible whole blood should be available, but need not be cross-matched until required.

A gentle enema before the operation will ensure that the rectum is empty which allows accurate palpation of the adenoma via the sterile urological drape and helps to protect the rectum from injury.

Operation

Equipment

Major transurethral surgery should be conducted in a properly equipped and maintained operating theatre which has adequate reserves of endoscopes, surgical diathermy units and light sources. Essential equipment includes a 19-Fr sheath with 0° telescope, 30° telescope and 70° telescope, 24-Fr and 27-Fr resectoscope sheaths, together with the appropriate working elements, cutting loops, button and ball electrodes. An Otis urethrotome, full range of urethral dilators, Ellick evacuator, Maryfield catheter introducer, three-way catheters for postoperative irrigation and copious supplies of sterile non-haemolysing irrigation fluid must be readily available. A sterile urological drape allows continuous monitoring of the progress of the operation by rectal palpation and helps to preserve the sterile operating field. Optional extras which may make the operation easier, safer and are desirable, range from the simple Iglesias continuous flow resectoscope to the elegant transducer-controlled low pressure continuous flow irrigation systems.

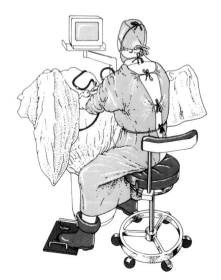

2 A microvideo operating system is invaluable to those with a heavy workload or teaching commitment.

2

Position of the patient

3 Positioning the patient is important. He may be immobilized for more than an hour and care should be taken to ensure there is no strain on his vulnerable hip and knee joints, and that pressure points are eliminated. This is best achieved by using purpose-built supports of the ski-boot variety and intermittent compression leg bags. A slight head-down tilt facilitates bladder perfusion.

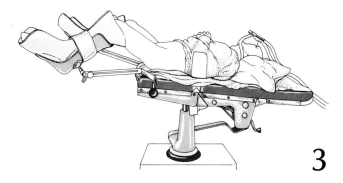

3

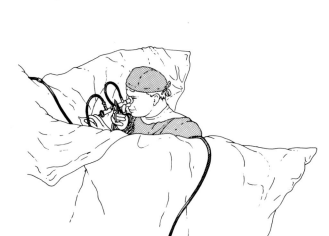

4

4 The comfort of the surgeon is equally important during a lengthy procedure and the technique of videoprostatectomy (or transurethral prostatectomy performed using a microvideo operating system) is recommended to reduce physical stress on the surgeon's spine and to allow him to operate with hands and arms in a natural position.

The magnified image on the video monitor aids tissue identification and reduces visual fatigue. The increased mobility of the resectoscope facilitates resection of anterior tissue and control of troublesome vessels. In patients with limited hip abduction, this technique will enable a transurethral operation to be performed which would otherwise be physically impossible. Finally the video technique removes the surgeon from intimate contact with the patient and helps protect him from contamination by blood-stained effluent.

Operative technique

5 Preliminary inspection of the well lubricated urethra by the 19-Fr endoscope with 0° telescope will identify abnormalities such as stricture, and permits initial evaluation of the prostate. The bladder is carefully examined with a 30° and 70° telescope to exclude associated pathology. The 24-Fr resectoscope sheath with Timberlake 'tilting-tip' obturator is gently passed. If there is resistance, Otis urethrotomy of the whole length of the urethra to 28 Fr will usually prevent postoperative stricture formation.

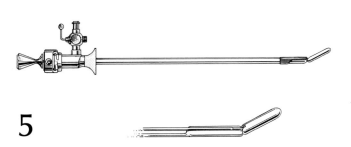

5

Attention is now focused on the prostate. There is surprising variation in the contour, size and vascularity of different glands. Each has its characteristics which should be evaluated both by inspection and by palpation through the rectum, with the resectoscope sheath *in situ*, using the sterile urological drape.

6 The verumontanum is the single most important landmark and must be clearly and readily identified. Cutting beyond this will damage the distal urethral closure mechanism and may result in permanent urinary incontinence.

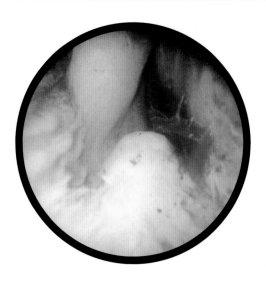

6

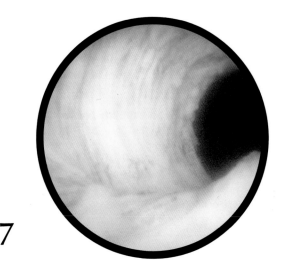

7

7 The circular fibres of the bladder neck are the other vital landmark and these should be carefully exposed at the beginning of the operation, usually starting in the 10 o'clock position and continuing around the entire circumference.

8 It may be necessary to trim down a prominent median lobe at this stage. This should be cut flush with the bladder neck. Particular care should be taken to avoid undermining the trigone which will create a flap which catches the beak of the resectoscope and may lead to significant fluid extravasation.

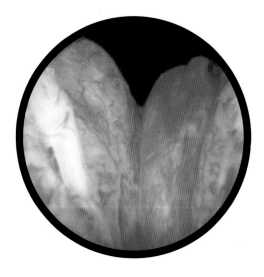

8

9 A trench is now cut in the 10 o'clock position down to the capsular fibres along the whole length of the right lateral lobe, constantly referring to the verumontanum as the distal landmark.

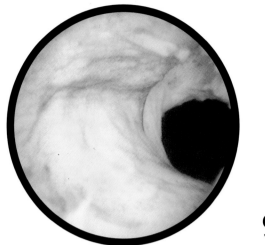

9

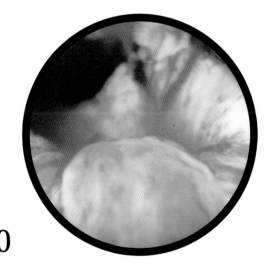

10

10 This allows the lateral lobe to fall down and across the midline which makes the subsequent resection easier, since the resectoscope will be cutting in the vertical position from the medial to lateral aspect of the lobe. The previously exposed bladder neck fibres are easily identified and prevent 'creeping down' the trigone.

11 The lateral lobe is progressively mobilized from the capsule until only apical tissue remains alongside the verumontanum. The remaining lateral lobe is removed in exactly the same way.

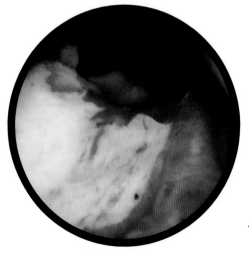

11

12 The two small apical areas are now removed safely by gently elevating them with a finger in the rectum.

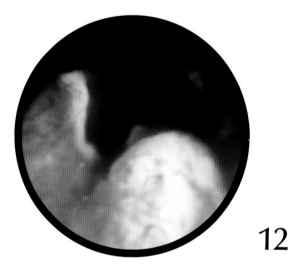

12

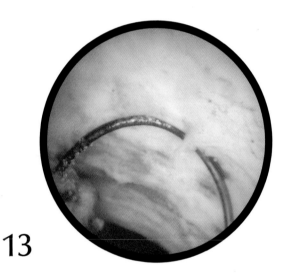

13

13 Residual anterior tissue, which may be very thin, is carefully trimmed to leave a clean, smooth, prostatic cavity.

14 The prostatic cavity is inspected for any remaining bleeding arteries which are sealed by pinpoint coagulation. Venous bleeding is similarly controlled. The main vessels which are usually situated in the 4 and 8 o'clock positions must be carefully secured.

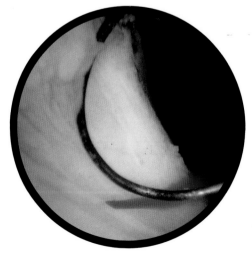

14

15 It is important to recognize capsular perforation which may lead to the opening of venous sinuses and extravasation. This frequently happens as a result of excessively deep resection through the thin anterolateral tissue. The appearance of filmy, cobweb tissue with fat or purple thin-walled sinuses bulging into the perforation is characteristic.

If a venous sinus has been breached, sudden heavy bleeding may obscure the view and it may be necessary to curtail the operation to prevent excessive blood loss or absorption of irrigant. Sinus bleeding can usually be controlled by tamponade with the balloon of the irrigation catheter; rarely is open surgical intervention required.

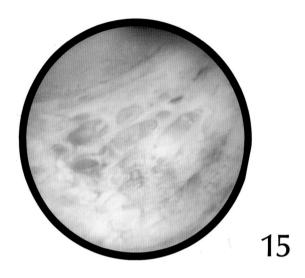

15

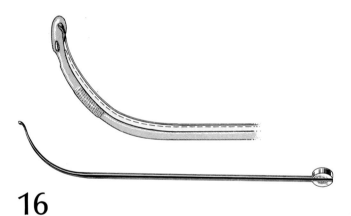

16

16 All the prostatic fragments are evacuated and if the patient's blood pressure has returned to a normal level, the resectoscope is removed and a three-way irrigation catheter is inserted using the Maryfield introducer which will prevent subtrigonal damage. The catheter is washed out several times until the effluent is clear and the surgeon is confident that there are no remaining prostatic fragments. After surgery an irrigation system is connected.

Postoperative care

The patient should be carefully monitored by experienced recovery room staff for the initial postoperative period. Pulse, blood pressure, oxygen saturation, irrigation inflow and outflow volumes, degree of haematuria, abdominal examination and temperature should all be recorded.

Irrigation and intravenous fluids should be pre-warmed to body temperature since patients may easily become relatively hypothermic with an adverse effect on the myocardium. Continuous flow irrigation is preferable to intermittent bladder washouts which breach the closed drainage system, but does require careful supervision lest the outflow becomes blocked and the bladder overdistended.

Intraoperative and postoperative blood loss may be difficult to assess when large volumes of irrigation fluid are involved. A dilutional colorimetric assessment of the effluent will give a good approximation, provided the total volume is accurately known.

A single dose of intravenous frusemide, 80 mg, may be helpful in combating early fluid overloading due to absorption through open venous sinuses, to promote renal function and to counteract hyponatraemia.

Most patients will not require whole blood transfusion. However, an experienced recovery room supervisor will rapidly alert the surgeon if postoperative bleeding does not rapidly respond to conservative methods such as light catheter traction. It is much easier and safer to return the patient to theatre from the recovery room if there is any doubt about haemostasis rather than to have to attempt to resuscitate a shocked patient with an emergency team in the middle of the night. The cavity can be washed out, inspected with the resectoscope and the offending vessels secured. Very rarely it may be necessary to resort to formal packing of the prostatic cavity.

Further complications should be rare after the patient returns to the ward. The urethral catheter is removed after 48 h and the patient is discharged when he has regained urinary control.

Outcome

Transurethral prostatectomy is a safe, comfortable and effective operation. The basic principles of the procedure are to ensure clear vision at all times, to secure haemostasis carefully as the operation proceeds, to maintain orientation by clearly identifying the verumontanum and circular bladder neck fibres throughout the course of the resection, and to recognize and evaluate capsular and sinus perforation.

Cold punch resection of the prostate

H. G. W. Frohmüller MD, MS, FACS
Professor and Chairman, Department of Urology, University of Würzburg Medical School, Würzburg, Germany

History

Transurethral resection of the prostate (TURP) by the cold punch technique is an alternative to electroresection. This method conforms with the fundamental principles of surgical technique. It causes minimal tissue trauma because the tissue is excised with a 'cold' knife, inflicting thermal destruction only in very small areas around bleeding vessels when haemostasis is applied by the tip of the coagulation electrode. The cold punch instrument is a direct vision endoscope that does not use a telescopic lens system during the resection process, thus allowing observation of the structures in their normal state, i.e. without magnification. As the lumen of the instrument is not narrowed by an electrotome, large quantities of irrigating fluid can pass freely, permitting clear vision even in the presence of bleeding.

In 1913 Young[1] published the development of the first punch instrument which permitted the removal of obstructive tissue at the posterior commissure without visualization. Braasch[2] improved this instrument in 1918 with his 'median bar excisor' which added direct vision to the punch procedure. Bumpus[3], like Braasch a urologist at the Mayo Clinic, solved the problem of haemorrhage in 1926 by designing an electrode-carrying guide. In 1935 Thompson[4], also at the Mayo Clinic, introduced his well-known cold punch resectoscope, which was universally employed without any major changes for the following 35 years. In 1972 Frohmüller[5] introduced a modification of the Thompson punch that is presently being used by most cold punch resectionists.

Principles and justification

1 The resectoscope consists of an outer sheath (a) with a built-in light-transmitting bundle and a connection for the light lead near the proximal end of the sheath. The cutting fenestra is located near the distal end. The adaptor (b) incorporates a large fluid outlet valve and an observation window with an air bubble eliminator. The central sheath (c) has a fluid inlet valve proximally and a tubular knife distally. An obturator (d) and a coagulation electrode (e) complete the instrument.

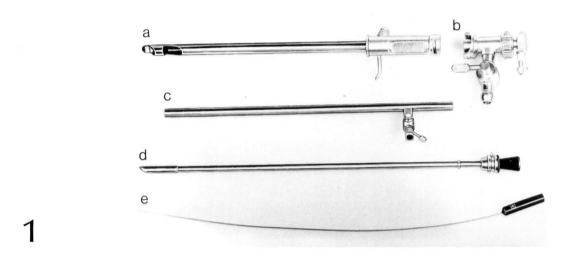

1

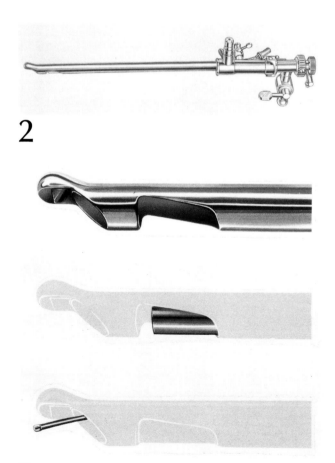

2

3

2, 3 The assembled instrument is used by moving the tubular knife distally.

Indications

The indications for performing cold punch resection for prostatic adenoma or carcinoma are no different from those for electroresection of the same conditions. Likewise, the basic principles of the operative technique of cold punch resection are much the same as those of electroresection.

At present, about 70% of all prostatectomies are being performed by transurethral resection. In our institution the ratio of cold punch resections *versus* open operations, i.e. suprapubic transvesical or retropubic extravesical, is about 95:5.

Contraindications

Diseases that limit movement of the patient's hip joints can be a contraindication to transurethral resection because of the necessity to put the patient on the operating table with his legs in abduction. Meatal stenosis and urethral stricture, however, do not constitute a contraindication because these conditions can be overcome by internal urethrotomy or a temporary perineal urethrotomy.

Preoperative

Preparation of the patient

The aim of preoperative care is to bring the patient to the optimum condition prior to undergoing transurethral resection. Coexisting diseases should be adequately treated and every effort should be made to keep the patient ambulatory during preoperative preparation.

Patients with impaired renal function may require preliminary drainage by an indwelling urethral catheter or a suprapubic cystostomy. Slow decompression of a chronically obstructed bladder is now considered unnecessary and may even be harmful.

Prophylactic bilateral vasectomy to reduce the risk of epididymitis is generally not necessary. The same beneficial effect can be achieved by a careful resection technique, avoiding injury to the verumontanum, and by adequate antimicrobial therapy.

Antimicrobial drugs for the prevention of urinary tract infection must be used cautiously. Patients with an acute infection should be given the appropriate drugs in therapeutic dosage.

Improvement of renal function and hydration is an important primary aim of preoperative care. Cardiovascular disease is rarely a contraindication to transurethral resection when modern anaesthesia is used. Any bleeding diathesis must be reversed prior to TURP.

Cross-matched whole blood or erythrocyte concentrate should be available during the transurethral procedure and in the immediate postoperative period.

The patient is a suitable candidate for transurethral resection when he is ambulatory, well nourished, well hydrated and mentally alert.

Anaesthesia

As for electroresection, spinal or epidural anaesthesia is used preferentially. This permits early detection of abdominal pain in the event of a perforation. Patients needing TURP are usually in the older age group. They tolerate a spinal anaesthetic better than a general anaesthetic and the former carries little risk of postoperative pulmonary complications.

Operation

Irrigating fluid

A non-haemolytic solution such as 3% sorbitol-mannitol or 1.1% glycine is used principally to prevent haemolytic reactions with resultant renal tubular insufficiency and anuria which occur when irrigating fluid enters the circulatory system via injured venous sinuses in the surgical capsule of the prostate.

Instruments

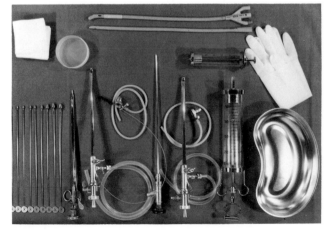

4 At the start of the resection the sterile instruments should be prepared on the instrument table. These should include an Otis bulb (Richard Wolf, Knittlingen, Germany) for urethral calibration, an Otis urethrotome, a telescope for viewing the bladder, a 24-Fr Couvelaire catheter (Willy Rüsch, Waiblingen, Germany) for irrigating the bladder, a 24-Fr three-way haemostatic catheter for postoperative bladder irrigation and a 50-ml syringe.

4

COLD PUNCH RESECTION

5 The punch instrument is introduced into the bladder in the same manner as an electroresectoscope. In the presence of a meatal stenosis or urethral stricture that is too narrow to admit easily the 28 Fr calibre of the punch instrument, an internal urethrotomy using the Otis urethrotome is performed. This simple procedure is necessary in about 40% of cases and will to a large degree prevent the development of postoperative strictures.

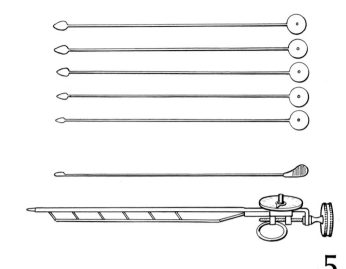

5

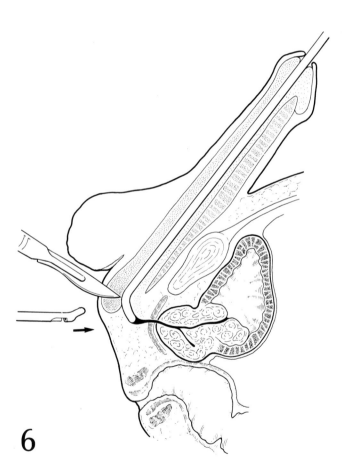

6

6 In the very rare case of a particularly long urethra the obstruction can be circumvented by a temporary perineal urethrotomy.

After the punch instrument has been introduced into the bladder, the obturator is withdrawn and the irrigating fluid inlet, the light cord and the electrode are connected. With the knife in the closed position and the fluid inlet open, the bladder, vesical neck and prostatic urethra are inspected. To avoid a collection of air bubbles or bloody fluid between the fluid inlet and the observation window, i.e. to keep the vision clear, the small outlet valve on the window should always remain open.

7 As the punch instrument does not incorporate an optical lens system, the objects are viewed without magnification and it is therefore necessary to change the position repeatedly in making a 360° excursion of the prostatic fossa. The knife is handled with the right hand. The convex surface of the outer sheath contains a fenestra close to the beak through which a tubular knife is advanced and withdrawn. In the forward position the cutting fenestra is closed. When the tubular knife is withdrawn, the cutting fenestra is opened to permit engagement of projecting prostatic tissue. The engaged tissue is cut off by punching the knife forward and washed into the bladder by the current of the irrigating fluid.

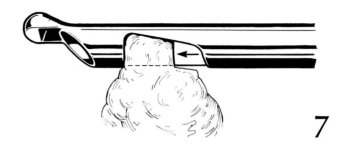

7

The inflow of fluid is controlled by the stop-cock on the knife element, which also serves as a thumb-rest. Beneath the proximal end of the outer sheath a large outlet is located. When this is opened and the fluid inlet closed, fluid from the bladder together with the resected tissue and blood clots is sucked off through an attached vacuum pump into a container. A wire strainer inside the glass container collects the resected tissue for histological examination. On the upper aspect of the outer sheath there is a small channel through which the coagulation electrode is passed. The knife must be kept razor sharp and should therefore be sharpened after one or two resections at the most.

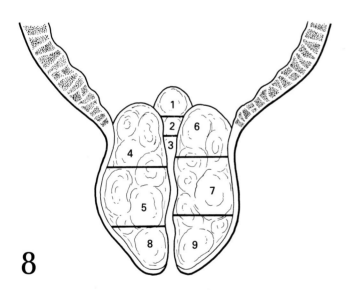

8

8 The sequence of resecting the obstructing prostatic tissue is illustrated. Modifications of this procedure may be necessary depending on the anatomy of the prostate in individual cases.

9 The tissue is identified visually as in electroresection. However, unlike the electroresectoscope, which does not permit the use of the surgeon's tactile sense, with the punch instrument the fibres of the vesical neck and the surgical capsule of the prostate tend to bind the knife, to adhere and to tear. Thus, injuries such as 'undermining the trigone' and perforation of the fibrous prostatic capsule can be more easily avoided. Palpation and pressure with the finger in the rectum is very helpful in identifying and excising residual adenomatous tissue.

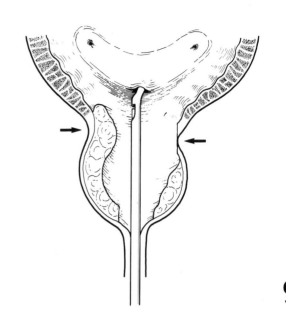

9

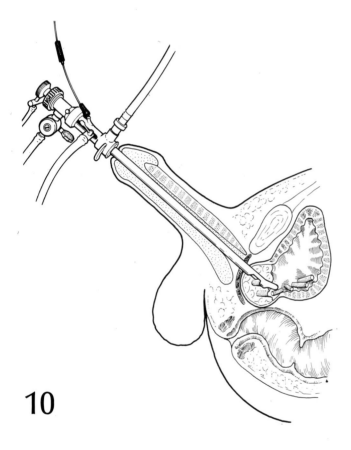

10

10 Bleeding is usually more profuse during punch resection than during electroresection, where some haemostasis is secured with the cutting current. It is a waste of time to coagulate bleeding vessels that are spurting from adenomatous tissue destined for excision. However, it is advisable to devote time to coagulating bleeding vessels when the fibrous capsule is reached. Minimal point coagulation should be employed to minimize thermal destruction of remaining tissue. As in electroresection it is futile to attempt to coagulate venous sinuses. This type of bleeding is best arrested by inflating a haemostatic catheter balloon in the prostatic fossa.

11 After careful coagulation and final inspection a three-way haemostatic irrigating catheter is introduced (usually 24 Fr) for continuous postoperative irrigation of the bladder with copious amounts of physiological saline. Parenchymatous bleeding can be well controlled by inflating the balloon in the prostatic fossa up to a volume of 20–100 ml. Continuous irrigation is routinely maintained for about 24 h.

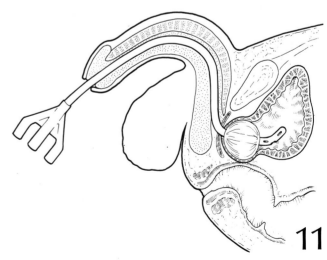

11

Postoperative care

Careful coagulation during resection and continuous irrigation will keep postoperative haemorrhage to a minimum. The continuous three-way irrigation system is preferable if significant bleeding is expected after the operation because the frequent blocking of the catheter with the associated necessity for frequent irrigation invites infection. Catheter traction is usually unnecessary. The haemostatic catheter is removed on the second or third postoperative day.

Whether or not it is beneficial to give antibiotics in the postoperative period has been a controversial subject for years. The development of postoperative bacteriuria and bacteraemia is often related to the presence of preoperative urinary tract infection. Prophylactic antimicrobials are mandatory for patients with valvular cardiac disease. Patients who do not have a preoperative urinary tract infection do not usually need prophylactic antibiotics after surgery.

When a non-haemolytic solution that minimizes the risk of intravascular haemolysis due to absorption of a hypotonic fluid such as water is used as irrigating fluid during resection, the transurethral resection (TUR) syndrome rarely occurs. It is caused by overhydration, which results in dilutional hyponatraemia due to the absorption of an excessive amount of irrigation fluid. The pressure in the prostatic venous plexus and pelvic veins is approximately 10 mmHg, thus any pressure within the prostatic urethra that is significantly higher than 10 mmHg leads to absorption when venous sinuses are opened. During an uncomplicated resection the average amount of irrigating fluid absorbed ranges from 100 ml to 1 litre. When larger quantities (up to 10 litres) are absorbed, the TUR syndrome ensues. Clinical symptoms usually occur when the serum sodium level falls below 120 mmol/l.

The clinical signs of the TUR syndrome depend on the type of anaesthesia used. The patient under spinal anaesthesia becomes restless and confused, complains of nausea, and develops hypertension and an increased venous pressure. Lower abdominal distension can occur. If pulmonary oedema develops, cyanosis and hypoxaemia associated with dyspnoea become apparent. In the unconscious patient under general anaesthesia the only signs are increasing systolic and diastolic pressure and an increased central venous pressure. Early recognition is the most important factor in the successful treatment of the TUR syndrome. This consists of the concomitant adminstration of hypertonic saline such as 250–500 ml of 3–5% sodium chloride and a diuretic such as frusemide, 40–100 mg, intravenously. Careful monitoring of the patient is mandatory.

Postoperative shock due to hypovolaemia as a result of intraoperative or postoperative bleeding requires the administration of blood transfusions. Careful postoperative monitoring of blood pressure and pulse rate are mandatory for the early recognition of hypotension with ensuing shock.

Cardiogenic shock due to pre-existing coronary artery disease may be triggered by hypovolaemia and electrolyte imbalance. It requires immediate treatment by an experienced team including a urologist, anaesthetist and nephrologist.

Septic shock is usually caused by infection of the urine with Gram-negative bacilli such as *Escherichia coli*, *Klebsiella* and *Pseudomonas*, acquired when the prostatic capsule was perforated with resulting extravasation of irrigation fluid. The patient develops fever, rigors, mental confusion and hypotension. Isotonic saline and whole blood infusion is indicated to replace volume loss, and broad-spectrum antibiotics are given intravenously. If pulmonary insufficiency (the so-called shock lung) occurs, intensive care and repeated intravenous injections of large doses of corticosteroids are required.

Outcome

The mortality rate following cold punch resection is similar to that following electroresection. In our institution the mortality rate during the last 10 years was 0.65%. There seems to be no age limit for cold punch resection or electroresection. They are equivalent procedures and both have advantages and disadvantages. Excellent results can be achieved by experienced urologists with the cold punch instrument as well as with the electroresectoscope.

References

1. Young HH. A new procedure (punch operation) for small prostatic bars and contracture of the prostatic orifice. *JAMA* 1913; 60: 253–7.

2. Braasch WF. Median bar excisor. *JAMA* 1918; 70: 758–9.

3. Bumpus HC. Results of punch prostatectomy. *J Urol* 1925; 16: 59–66.

4. Thompson GJ. A new direct vision resectoscope. *Urol Cutan Rev* 1935; 39: 545–6.

5. Frohmüller HGW. Direktsichtinstrumente in der Urologie. *Verh Dtsch Ges Urol* 1973: 331–4.

Further reading

Emmett JL. Transurethral resection with the cold punch: operative technique. *J Urol* 1943; 49: 815–39.

Frohmüller HGW. An improved cold punch resectoscope. *Endoscopy* 1976; 8: 195–8.

Frohmüller HGW. Transurethral resection of the prostate by cold punch technique. In: Fitzpatrick JM, Krane RJ, eds. *The Prostate*. Edinburgh: Churchill Livingstone, 1989: 237–43.

Nation EF. Evolution of knife-punch resectoscope. *Urology* 1976; 7: 417–27.

Illustrations by Paul Richardson

Balloon dilatation of the prostatic urethra

Gordon Williams MS, FRCS
Consultant Urologist, Hammersmith Hospital, London and Honorary Senior Lecturer, Royal Postgraduate Medical School, London, UK

John McLoughlin MS, FRCS
Urological Registrar, Hammersmith Hospital, London, UK

History

Balloon dilatation of the prostatic urethra to relieve bladder outflow obstruction is an extension of the work of Mercier in 1844. His metal dilator was modified by Deisting in 1950 with an immediate success of 95% and a symptomatic recurrence rate of 15% at 8 years. Balloon dilatation of the prostatic urethra was first successfully described by Burhenne et al. in 1984[1] and has subsequently found considerable popularity in North America, but the majority of studies base their results on little more than symptomatic improvement or flow rate analysis.

Principles and justification

Indications

Men with urodynamic evidence of bladder outflow obstruction with a gland size of less than 40 g assessed by ultrasonography and with no significant middle lobe enlargement are most likely to respond. There is no role for balloon dilatation in patients presenting with acute or chronic retention of urine[2].

Preoperative

The presence of bladder outflow obstruction should be confirmed by urodynamic investigations. The dilatation can be performed on a day-case basis. A broad-spectrum antibiotic is administered intravenously immediately before the procedure. The patient is sedated with intravenous midazolam and pethidine hydrochloride.

Operation

The patient is placed in the lithotomy position and a preliminary cystourethroscopy is performed under general anaesthesia.

Two types of balloon are in common use. The ASI Uroplasty balloon (Advanced Surgical Intervention, California, USA) is a high-pressure triple-lumen balloon catheter, which can be inflated to 75 Fr at a pressure of 3 atm and is inserted under direct cystoscopic control.

1 The distance from the bladder neck to the external sphincter is measured endoscopically following the passage of a graduated balloon occlusion catheter. A Uroplasty prostatic dilatation catheter is chosen to match this length.

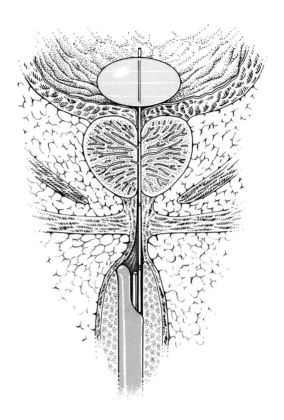

1

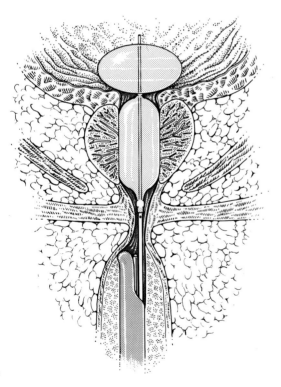

2

2 The catheter is passed through the cystoscope and the distal balloon inflated; the catheter is then withdrawn so that the balloon lodges on the bladder neck. The metallic marker on the catheter should now lie at the level of the external sphincter. The position of the metallic marker can be checked either endoscopically or by digital rectal palpation.

Keeping traction on the catheter and ensuring endoscopically that there is no migration of the catheter into the bladder, the pressurized balloon is inflated to a pressure of 3 atmospheres maintained for 15 min. The balloons are then deflated, and the catheter and endoscope removed. A 14-Fr Foley catheter is left in the bladder for 24 h.

3 Single balloon catheters are available in sizes 20–35 Fr. Better results have been reported with the larger balloons. A preliminary cystourethroscopy is performed. A guidewire is inserted along the sheath of the cystoscope and the balloon inserted over the wire. Under direct vision, the balloon is positioned by aligning the metal ring at the distal extremity of the balloon just proximal to the external sphincter. Considerable traction has to be maintained on the catheter to prevent it migrating into the bladder while inflated. The dilatation lasts for 15 min and a 14-Fr Foley catheter is inserted for 24 h.

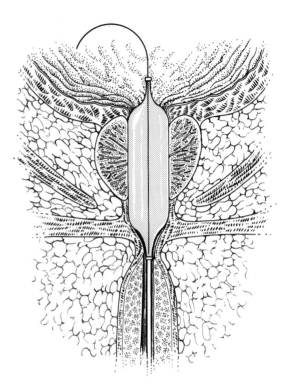

3

Postoperative care

The patient is allowed home with the indwelling catheter *in situ*. This is removed after 24 h. Transient haematuria occurs in most patients, and in some it may be necessary to leave the catheter *in situ* for 48 h.

Long-term follow-up is essential. Although 80% of men can be expected to improve symptomatically, objective evidence of improvement at 1 year is far less common.

References

1. Burhenne HJ, Chisholm RJ, Quenville F. Prostatic hyperplasia: radiological intervention. Work in progress. *Radiology* 1984; 152: 655–7.

2. McLoughlin J, Keane PF, Jager R, Gill KP, Machann L, Williams G. Dilatation of the prostatic urethra with 35 mm balloon. *Br J Urol* 1991; 67: 177–81.

Prostatic stents

Gordon Williams MS, FRCS
Consultant Urologist, Hammersmith Hospital, London and Honorary Senior Lecturer, Royal Postgraduate
Medical School, London, UK

John McLoughlin MS, FRCS
Urological Registrar, Hammersmith Hospital, London, UK

History

Since the 16th century, metallic implants have been used with variable success as prosthetic and therapeutic surgical devices. Metallic prostatic stents are of two types:

1. Permanently implanted prostatic stents[1] consisting of an expandable stainless steel or titanium mesh (through which the urothelium grows to cover the stent permanently).
2. Removable intraprostatic spirals[2].

Principles and justification

Indications

Over 150 permanently implanted stents have now been inserted by our group to relieve bladder outflow obstruction secondary to prostatic disease, but follow-up is limited[1,3]. Initially, stents were inserted in men with proven bladder outflow obstruction who were unfit for surgery and in whom the alternative treatment would have been insertion of a permanent indwelling urethral catheter. With greater experience, these stents are now being offered to men who would otherwise undergo prostatectomy.

Prostatic spirals are an alternative to an indwelling catheter for patients awaiting prostatic surgery. They may be used with less success in those who are unfit or unwilling to undergo prostatic surgery. They may also be used in patients with neurological disorders or cerebral impairment to determine whether they are likely to remain continent if a prostatectomy is performed.

Preoperative

The procedure is carried out on an inpatient basis. The patient is given broad-spectrum antibiotic prophylaxis for 24 h, commencing before stent insertion. The patient is sedated with intravenous midazolam and pethidine.

Operation

PERMANENTLY IMPLANTED STENTS

The patient is placed in the lithotomy position. A cystourethroscopy is performed. The distance between the bladder neck and the verumontanum is measured using a graduated balloon occlusion catheter, and a stent of appropriate length is chosen. With a large prostate, it may be necessary to insert two stents.

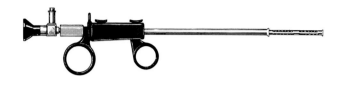

1 The AMS Urolume stent (American Medical Systems, Lausanne, Switzerland) comes with its own endoscopic delivery device.

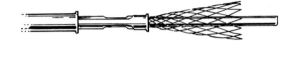

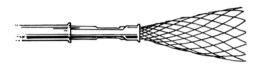

1

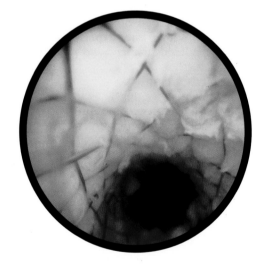

2

2 Using a 0° telescope, the bladder neck is visualized and the stent slowly released so that its proximal end just overlies the bladder neck. The position of the stent is checked repeatedly during its release. The safety catch of the delivery device is only released when the stent can be seen to extend from the bladder neck to the verumontanum.

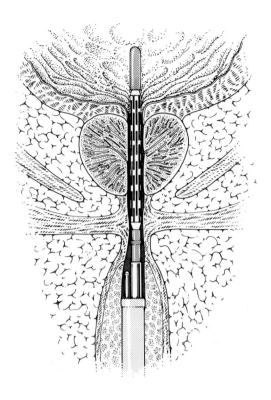

3,4 The ASI stent (Advanced Surgical Intervention, California, USA) is mounted on a deflated balloon catheter and is inserted under direct vision with a cystoscope. When it is in the correct position, with the proximal end just overlying the bladder neck and the distal end over the verumontanum, the balloon is inflated to expand the stent. When the stent is in position the balloon is deflated and removed.

If the stents are accidentally released or dislodged into the bladder, the manufacturer provides a grasping device to remove the stent.

If the prostatic urethra is too long for a single stent, the proximal stent is inserted first and a second distal stent inserted so that its proximal end interdigitates with the distal end of the first stent.

3

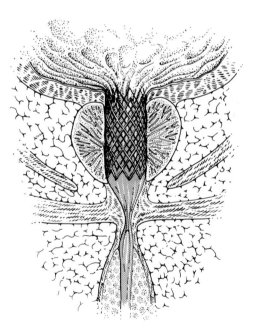

4

INTRAPROSTATIC SPIRALS

5 A preliminary cystourethroscopy should be carried out on all patients. The length of the prostatic urethra is measured as when inserting a permanently implanted stent.

A spiral 10–15 mm longer than this is chosen to ensure that the tip projects into the bladder. A 7-Fr ureteric catheter is passed into the bladder and the spiral is mounted on it and pushed into position. Its position can be checked either endoscopically or ultrasonographically.

If the spiral needs to be removed, this should be attempted endoscopically with the aid of a ureteric balloon occlusion catheter passed through the spiral. The balloon is inflated and the spiral is withdrawn mounted on the catheter. Simply grasping the catheter with forceps causes it to unspiral and elongate considerably so that the urethra can be traumatized.

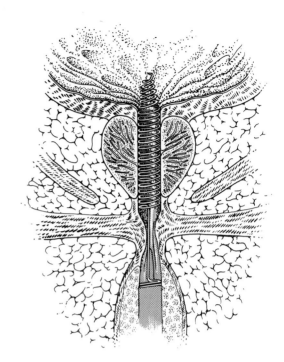

5

Postoperative care

If the patient is unable to void, a suprapubic catheter must be inserted. Any urethral instrumentation during the first 6 weeks following stent insertion is likely to dislodge the stent into the bladder.

Complications

Severe frequency and urgency of micturition with occasional incontinence are common during the first 3–4 days and gradually resolve over 3–4 weeks.

Most patients have infected urine at the time of stent insertion. This usually resolves without antibiotics once the stent has epithelialized and the patient is voiding and emptying his bladder. If the stent is incorrectly placed, e.g. if part is projecting into the bladder, these areas will not epithelialize. Calcification and stone formation on these areas has been reported with the AMS stent. Ingrowth of urothelium can occur, but seldom obstructs the flow of urine. This ingrowth can easily be resected using a standard resectoscope.

The intraprostatic spirals do not epithelialize and may dislocate proximally or distally, requiring either readjustment of their position or removal. Calcification and persistent infection are fairly common, as is perineal discomfort and haematuria. Persistence of these complaints necessitates removal of the spiral.

References

1. Williams G. Early experience of the use of permanently implanted prostatic stents for the treatment of bladder outflow obstruction. *World J Urol* 1991; 9: 26–8.

2. Nielsen KK, Klarsov P, Nordling J, Andersen JT, Holm HH. The intraprostatic spiral. New treatment for urinary retention. *Br J Urol* 1990; 65: 500–3.

3. Williams G, Jager R, McLoughlin J *et al*. Use of stents for treating obstruction of urinary outflow in patients unfit for surgery. *BMJ* 1989; 298: 1429.

Hyperthermia of the prostate for benign prostatic hyperplasia

Claude C. Schulman MD, PhD
Professor of Urology, University Clinics of Brussels, Erasme Hospital, Brussels, Belgium

Marc Vandenbossche MD
Urologist, University Clinics of Brussels, Erasme Hospital, Brussels, Belgium

The currently accepted treatment for obstructive benign prostatic hyperplasia (BPH) is transurethral resection of the prostate or open prostatectomy. Clear indications for surgery are limited to chronic retention or recurrent urinary infection or renal failure due to BPH. The majority of patients, however, complain of a train of symptoms called prostatism and do not necessarily need surgery. This is probably the group for whom non-surgical treatment of BPH is appropriate. Alpha-blockers, androgen deprivation and especially 5α-reductase inhibitors, balloon dilatation and hyperthermia are alternatives to surgery but their indications must be specified. During the last few years, much effort has been devoted to developing prostatic hyperthermia technology for use in the treatment of BPH.

History, principles and justification

The first effect of heating tissue was described by Busch[1] in 1866. He related a case of a histologically proven sarcoma which disappeared completely following a febrile attack caused by erysipelas. Tumour cells are more sensitive to heating than are normal cells and seem to be killed by temperatures ranging from 42°C to 44°C. Benign cells are affected at 44–45°C[2]. The most important factor is probably defective heat dissipation by the neoplastic tissue due to poor blood supply and decreased vasodilatory capacity of the neovascular bed in response to a rise in temperature. Hyperthermic toxicity is time and temperature dependent. Hyperthermia is recognized as an effective potentiating adjuvant when used in conjunction with radiation and/or chemotherapeutic agents for the treatment of malignant disease[3]. Local hyperthermia of the prostate utilizes temperatures ranging from 42°C to 45°C. Thermotherapy uses temperatures ranging from 45°C to 55°C to cause necrosis of benign prostatic tissue.

Local hyperthermia can be produced using either microwave radiation of different frequencies or radiofrequencies transmitted by special applicators[4]. The area heated is determined by the size and shape of the applicator while the depth of heating, which is a function of wavelength and the electric properties of the tissues, is controlled by the choice of frequency.

Several hyperthermia or thermotherapy devices are now available and the majority use microwaves originating from a transurethral or transrectal probe. One device uses radiofrequency waves from a transurethral source.

Indications

Prostatic hyperthermia is indicated in the following:

1. Patients with contraindications to transurethral resection of the prostate or adenomectomy.
2. Patients with symptomatic prostatism hoping essentially for a subjective improvement.
3. Patients with chronic retention (transurethral hyperthermia has about a 40% success rate) wishing to delay an operation or, in some instances, to avoid it[5].

Contraindications

Poor results have been reported in patients with obstruction from middle lobe prostatic enlargement. The following are contraindications to prostatic hyperthermia:

1. Urethral stricture.
2. Prostatic neoplasm.
3. Previous prostatic surgery.

4. Urinary tract infection at the time of treatment.
5. Total hip replacement or the presence of other pelvic or femoral implants.
6. Pacemakers.
7. Evidence of blood coagulation disorder.

Preoperative

Patients are treated on an outpatient basis. Before treatment they are investigated by uroflowmetry and transrectal prostatic ultrasonography and are examined carefully with regard to residual urine and absence of prostatic cancer. A subjective symptom score is used for assessment.

Equipment

The available transrectal and transurethral devices are compared in *Tables 1* and *2* respectively.

The transrectal approach uses a probe that emits the waves together with a cooling system to protect the rectal wall. A urethral catheter is inserted to monitor the temperature in the prostatic urethra in the Prostathermer machine (Biodan Medical Systems, Rehovot, Israel) while in the transrectal Primus machine (Tecnomatix, Antwerp, Belgium) the temperature is estimated by a computer.

The Thermex II (Direx Systems, Petah-Tikva, Israel) and BSD (BSD Medical Corporation, Salt Lake City, USA) transurethral devices use only transurethral catheters with a transurethral applicator whereas the Prostatron (Technomed, Paris, France) requires in addition a

Table 1   Transrectal hyperthermia devices for benign prostatic hyperplasia

	Prostathermer	Primus
Single session	No	No
Rectal probe	Yes	Yes
Simultaneous treatment	No	No
Cooling system	Yes	Yes
Wavelength (MHz)	915	915

Table 2 Transurethral hyperthermia devices for benign prostatic hyperplasia

	Thermex-II	BSD	Prostatron
Single session	Yes	No	Yes
Rectal probe	No	No	Yes
Simultaneous treatment	Yes	No	No
Cooling system	No	No	Yes
Wavelength (MHz)	Radiofrequency Mixture of waves	434	1296

transurethral cooling system and a rectal probe to monitor the rectal temperature.

All the devices, apart from the Prostatron, are mobile and can be used in any room selected by the physician. The Prostatron needs a special room because it is cumbersome and the patient has to lie on it.

Anaesthesia

The only anaesthesia required is intraurethral lignocaine jelly. If treatment becomes painful, intravenous sedation with diazepam or pethidine may be necessary.

Postoperative care

Patients are given a urinary antiseptic and a non-steroidal anti-inflammatory drug for several days after treatment. They may suffer from a temporary deterioration of urinary performance or from acute retention for which temporary bladder drainage (transurethral or suprapubic) is necessary. Patients are followed up with the same urodynamic evaluations as before treatment.

Outcome

Assessment is clouded by the number of different devices that have been developed with various treatment regimens. Results are mostly reported in terms of symptom scores and are therefore subjective. They remain somewhat controversial.

The transrectal route essentially provides subjective improvement: in two placebo-controlled studies one showed a small difference between the treated group and the control group and the other showed no significant change in objective criteria between the groups[6-11].

With the transurethral approach, subjective improvement is obtained in 60–70% of patients, depending on the series and the device used. The objective increase in peak flow is variable and depends on the selection of patients. Those with a starting peak flow of less than 10 ml/s seem to respond best.

About 40% of patients with chronic retention become catheter-free after transurethral hyperthermia treatment[12, 13].

Mode of action

Glandular and smooth muscle cell necrosis have been demonstrated after transurethral hyperthermia and transurethral thermotherapy as deep as 2 cm from the urethra. Tissue necrosis may lead to urethral decompression and diminution of urethral resistance with improvement in flow. Hyperthermia may also induce neuromuscular lesions with destruction of α-receptors at the bladder neck and in the prostatic urethra which may explain the reduction of irritative symptoms such as urgency, frequency and nocturia[5, 12–14].

Complications

Transient voiding difficulties may occur. Acute retention develops in 10–20% of patients depending on the equipment used. Urethral pain, haematuria and urinary tract infection may also arise.

Conclusion

This new treatment of symptomatic BPH is still controversial. Results lack long-term follow-up and are expressed in different ways. The exact efficacy of this treatment of BPH remains uncertain and appears at the present time to provide essentially only subjective improvement. It should be regarded as a possible treatment option in selected patients to improve symptoms subjectively or in patients with inoperable obstructive BPH.

Hyperthermia may change clinical prostatism to silent prostatism, to the satisfaction of the patient if not to the urologist.

References

1. Busch W. Uber den Einflusse welchen heltigere Erysipeln zuweiten auf organisierte neubildungen. *Verh Naturheid Preuss Rhein Westphal* 1866; 23: 28–30.

2. Cavaliere R, Ciocatto EC, Clovanelle BC *et al*. Selective heat sensitivity of cancer cells: biochemical and clinical studies. *Cancer* 1967; 20: 1351–81.

3. Kim SH, Kim JH, Hahn EW. The enhanced killing of irradiated Hela cells in synchronous culture by hyperthermia. *Radiat Res* 1976; 66: 337–45.

4. Leveen HH. Radiofrequency in the treatment of malignant tumours. *Topical Rev Radiother Oncol* 1982; 2: 129–73.

5. Schulman CC, van den Bossche M. Transurethral hyperthermia and PSA markers. *J Endourol* 1991; 5(Suppl 1): S88.

6. Lindner A, Braf Z, Lev A *et al*. Local hyperthermia of the prostate gland for the treatment of benign prostatic hypertrophy and urinary retention. *Br J Urol* 1990; 65: 201–3.

7. Servadio C, Braf Z, Siegel Y, Leib Z, Saranga R, Lindner A. Local thermotherapy of the benign prostate. A 1-year follow-up. *Eur Urol* 1990; 18: 169–73.

8. Strohmaier WL, Bichler KH, Flüchter SH, Wilbert DM. Local microwave hyperthermia of benign prostatic hyperplasia. *J Urol* 1990; 144: 913–17.

9. Watson GM, Perlmutter AP, Shah TK, Barnes DG. Heat treatment for severe, symptomatic prostatic outflow obstruction. *World J Urol* 1991; 9: 7–11.

10. Yerushalmi A, Fishelovitz Y, Singer D *et al*. Localized deep microwave hyperthermia in the treatment of poor operative risk patients with benign prostatic hyperplasia. *J Urol* 1985; 133: 873–6.

11. Zerbib M, Steg A, Conquy S, Debré B. A prospective randomized study of localized hyperthermia versus placebo in obstructive benign hypertrophy of the prostate. *J Urol* 1990; 143(Suppl): 284A (Abstract 383).

12. Devonec M, Berger N, Bringeon G, Carter S, Perrin P. Long-term results of transurethral microwave therapy (TUMT) in patients with benign prostatic hypertrophy. *J Urol* 1991; 145: 390A (Abstract 709).

13. van den Bossche M, Noël JC, Schulman CC. Transurethral hyperthermia for benign prostatic hypertrophy. *World J Urol* 1991; 9: 2–6.

14. Leib Z, Rothem A, Lev A, Servadio C. Histopathological observation in the canine prostate treated by local microwave hyperthermia. *Prostate* 1986; 8: 93–102.

Illustrations by Peter Cox

Laparoscopic pelvic lymph node dissection

L. G. Gomella MD
Assistant Professor, Department of Urology, Jefferson Medical College, Thomas Jefferson University, Philadelphia, Pennsylvania, USA

M. Kozminski MD
Phoenix Urology Institute, St Joseph, Missouri, USA

History

The first reported use of laparoscopy was in 1911 when a cystoscope was used to examine the abdomen in a patient with ascites[1]. Since that first effort, advances in light sources, lens systems, operating instruments and techniques have made operative laparoscopy and 'minimally' invasive endosurgery a reality. Gynaecologists have been the leaders in the application of laparoscopy, and recently surgeons in other disciplines are realizing the potential benefits of laparoscopy.

Although laparoscopy has been used in urology (such as in the localization of undescended testicles), transperitoneal lymph node dissection for staging prostate and bladder cancer, varicocoele ligation, biopsy of pelvic masses and lymphocoele drainage are all new uses of the technique. Carcinoma of the prostate is the most prevalent solid tumour in American men, so laparoscopic pelvic lymph node dissection as a staging tool currently has the most widespread appeal.

Laparoscopic lymph node dissection has several advantages over conventional open pelvic lymph node dissection, including shorter hospitalization (2 days compared with 5 days), quicker resumption of normal activities (1 week compared with 4 weeks), less pain and overall lower cost. Preliminary studies indicate that the number of pelvic lymph nodes removed with the laparoscope is similar to that removed by open lymph node dissection.

Principles and justification

Indications

Because this is a relatively new procedure, the absolute indications and contraindications are not yet firmly established. Clearly, not all patients with prostate cancer need to be staged with a laparoscopic pelvic lymph node dissection. At present, the procedure is most useful in those patients thought to have classification 'D1' prostate cancer (pelvic node involvement) but where this cannot be determined conclusively by other less invasive studies, or where definitive therapy such as radiation therapy is being considered and accurate staging of the nodes is critical.

Contraindications

Potential contraindications include the inability to tolerate a general anaesthetic or pneumoperitoneum (due to heart or lung disease), extreme obesity, large intra-abdominal masses, ileus or obstruction, extensive lower abdominal surgery, aneurysmal disease, previous vascular graft surgery, inflammatory bowel disease, history of peritonitis and diaphragmatic hernia.

Preoperative

Patients are given a mild bowel preparation (magnesium hydroxide the afternoon before and a Fleet enema (sodium phosphate and sodium acid phosphate) the morning of the procedure). Patients are also encouraged to avoid dairy products for 2 days before the procedure, to help control intestinal gas. Broad-spectrum prophylactic antibiotics (such as ceftriaxone) are given before the operation and after surgery in a dose of 1 g 12-hourly for two doses. Intermittent pneumatic compression stockings are applied to help prevent deep venous thrombosis.

Laparoscopic instrumentation used in interventional gynaecology or in laparoscopic cholecystectomy is easily adapted to laparoscopic lymph node dissection. It is advisable also to have a laparotomy set-up available in case it is needed. Two operating surgeons and a camera assistant, in addition to the usual scrub nurse and circulating nurse, are needed. The operation is viewed by all parties on a video monitor and the importance of close team work cannot be overemphasized.

Anaesthesia

General anaesthesia is administered endotracheally and a nasogastric tube and Foley catheter are placed. Nitrous oxide anaesthesia is discouraged since it can cause bowel distension.

Operation

The patient is positioned supine with a roll of towels under the buttocks, and the table is broken slightly to allow easier access to the pelvis. The entire abdomen, from pubis to the subcostal area, is prepared. Gentle Trendelenburg positioning will displace the small intestine out of the operative field. Rolling the table to the opposite side of the dissection also helps improve visualization by moving the intestines out of the field.

1 Four operative ports are usually used

A small incision is made at the base of the umbilicus down to the fascia. The abdominal wall is lifted upward, usually with the aid of towel clips placed on either side of the umbilicus, and a Veress needle is passed through the fascia and into the abdominal cavity. The spring-loaded tip of the needle helps prevent inadvertent bowel injury. A water test is then performed to verify the needle is inside the peritoneum: 5–10 ml of water is injected into the needle and an attempt made to aspirate the water; if the needle is in the correct position, the water cannot be aspirated. False positive tests can be seen, however; if the initial pressure of the pneumoperitoneum is below 6–8 mmHg, the needle is probably in the peritoneal cavity.

Next, the pneumoperitoneum is created. The Veress needle is connected to the CO_2 insufflator and approximately 4–5 litres at 12–15 mmHg pressure are introduced. Insufflation of the abdomen is monitored by percussing over the right hypochondrium; a dull echo tone indicates proper insufflation. The high-flow insufflator should maintain pressure at approximately 15 mmHg. A high-flow insufflator capable of flow rates of 3–10 l/min is essential to maintain an adequate pneumoperitoneum.

The Veress needle is removed and the 10 or 10/11 mm trocar is passed into the abdominal cavity. (Newer disposable trocars have a retractable safety shield that covers the sharp needle tip after it enters the abdomen.) The laparoscope is placed in this umbilical port, the video camera attached and a brief visual inspection of the abdomen performed. The remaining trocars are inserted under direct vision. A 10 or

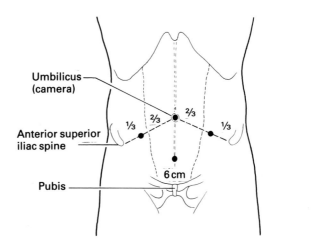

10/11 mm trocar is placed approximately 6–7 cm above the pubic ramus and two 5 mm trocars are placed in the right and left lower quadrants just lateral to the rectus muscles at a point approximately midway between the umbilicus and anterior superior iliac spine. The choice of size of the ports is up to the operator; some prefer to use 10 or 10/11 mm trocars laterally and a 5 mm port medially. We prefer the larger port in the midline so that larger instruments, such as clip appliers and specimen extractors, can be easily used on either the right or left side. Trocar insertion should be visualized to help prevent injury to the epigastric vessels laterally.

Fogging of the lens can be dealt with easily by touching the lens on the bowel; touching fat will usually leave a film on the lens. Anti-fog solutions and newer self-cleaning laparoscopes are also available. The right-sided node dissection is usually performed first, with the primary surgeon on the patient's left and the assistant on the right. For the left-sided dissection, the primary surgeon stands on the right side. The video monitor is placed near the patient's feet.

2 The key landmarks at the pelvic side wall are visualized through the peritoneum: they are the medial umbilical ligament (obliterated umbilical artery), epigastric vessels, vas deferens, internal inguinal ring, external iliac vessels and the spermatic vessels. In most patients the ureter can be seen more proximally as it crosses the iliac vessels. The position of the ureter should be rechecked before removing the proximal external iliac lymph node tissue.

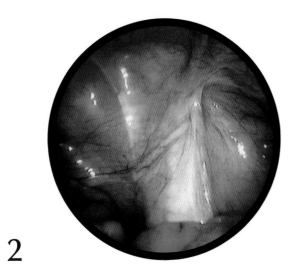

2

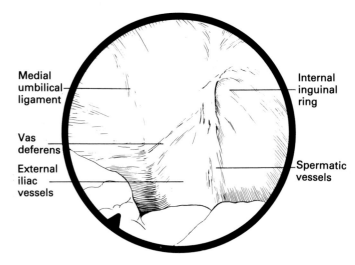

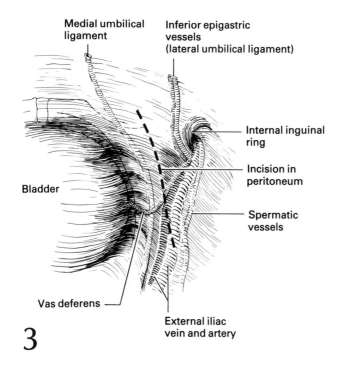

3

3 The limits of the dissection are identical to those for open pelvic lymph node dissection for prostate cancer. For purposes of staging prostate cancer, the so called 'limited obturator' lymph node dissection is used. The dissection begins using the umbilical ligament as the initial landmark. This structure defines the medial extent of the dissection. With medium traction on the ligament, a longitudinal incision is made in the peritoneal reflection just lateral to the ligament at the approximate level of the internal inguinal ring, across the vas and gently curving laterally in the direction of the bifurcation of the iliac vessels. The authors prefer the NdYAG contact laser (set at 10 W continuous power) for the incision.

4 The peritoneum is opened and the vas deferens identified as it crosses the middle of the incision. The vas is clipped with haemoclips and transected with the laser or scissors. This allows maximal medial retraction of the umbilical ligament.

At the distal end of the incision the pubic ramus is identified, initially by feeling for the bone and then visually after the loose fibroareolar tissue is gently stripped. Often accessory vessels are found that require careful dissection or the use of a haemoclip.

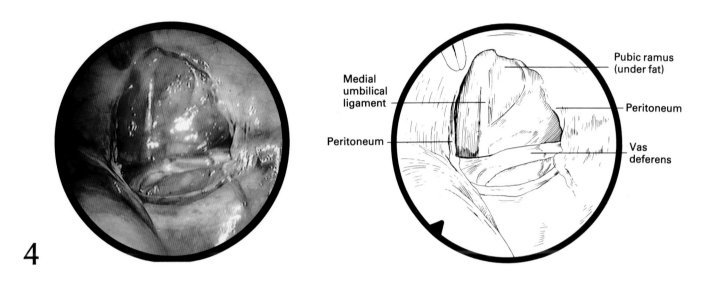

4

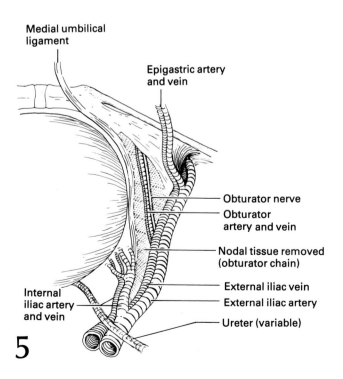

5

5 The tissue should be swept medially using blunt dissection until the obturator nerve and vessels are identified medially and the external iliac vein is seen laterally. Effective counter-traction makes the dissection easier. A specimen of the nodal tissue between the obturator nerve and external iliac vein is taken. The dissection continues medially along the umbilical ligament, proximally to the point where the obturator nerve, umbilical ligament and external iliac vein meet and laterally along the external iliac vein. The ureter should be noted as it crosses the vessels more proximally; the obturator node dissection is always distal to the ureter.

6 Proximal dissection may be difficult since the internal iliac vein often can not be well visualized. The nodal packet may then be removed either in a block or in separate segments through the 10 or 10/11 port.

A suction/irrigation device is used to inspect for any bleeding sites.

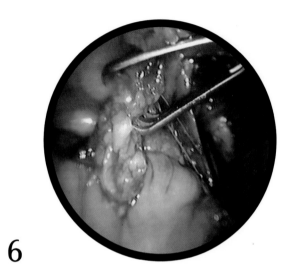

6

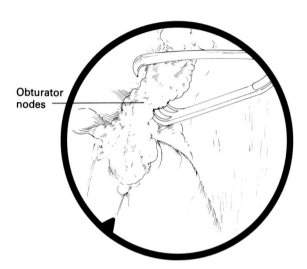

Obturator nodes

7 A completed right-sided dissection is shown. It is the authors' practice to submit any clinically suspicious nodes for frozen section analysis at this point.

If the nodes demonstrate tumour involvement, the procedure is usually terminated.

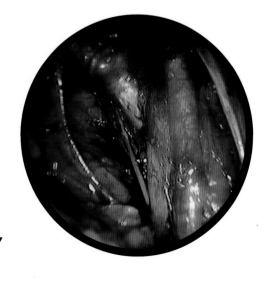

7

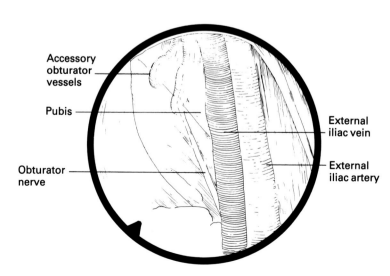

Accessory obturator vessels

Pubis

Obturator nerve

External iliac vein

External iliac artery

8   The left-sided dissection is completed in a similar fashion. Sigmoid adhesions often occur on the left side, but are easily taken down with the contact NdYAG laser or scissors. In all other aspects, the dissections are identical.

At the end of the procedure, the trocars are removed, visually inspecting for bleeding with the laparoscope as they leave the abdomen. The laparoscopic port is the last to be removed and as much CO_2 as possible should be expelled from the abdomen. Smaller (5 mm) trocar insertion sites are closed with absorbable suture; for the 10 or 10/11 trocar sites fascial closure is made with 2/0 absorbable suture and absorbable suture for the skin.

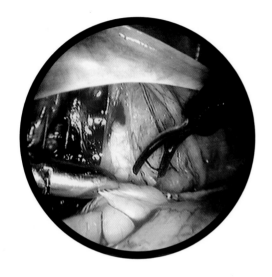

8

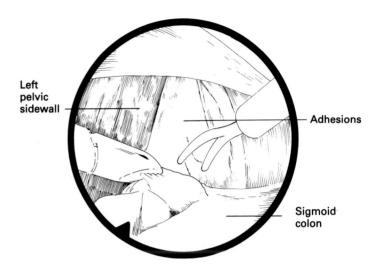

Left pelvic sidewall

Adhesions

Sigmoid colon

Postoperative care

Patients are usually allowed clear liquids within several hours of surgery and quickly advanced to a regular diet. Most patients are discharged within 24–48 h of the procedure and return to full activities after 1 week.

Complications

Reported complications include: bleeding; inadvertent bowel, bladder or ureteric injury; equipment failure; atelectasis; and other complications of general anaesthesia. Complications unique to laparoscopic surgery (related to the CO_2-induced pneumoperitoneum) can include subcutaneous emphysema, pneumoscrotum, hypercarbia and hypothermia. Lymphocoele formation is not usually seen with laparoscopic lymphadenectomy since the bed of the dissection is open to the peritoneum.

References

1. Jacobeus HC. Kurze Ubersicht meine Erfahrungen mit de Laparoskopie. *Munch Med Wochenschr* 1911; 58: 2017–19.

Further reading

Elder JS. Laparoscopy and Fowler–Stephens orchiopexy in the management of the impalpable testis. *Urol Clin North Am* 1989; 16: 399–411.

Scheussler WW, Vanciallie TG, Reich H, Griffith DP. Transperitoneal endosurgical lymphadenectomy in patients with localized prostate cancer. *J Urol* 1991; 145: 988–91.

Winfield HN. Suddenly, urology takes up the laparoscope. *Contemp Urol* 1991; 3: 70–80.

Cystourethroscopy

H. N. Whitfield MA, MChir, FRCS
Consultant Urologist, St Bartholomew's Hospital and St Mark's Hospital for Diseases of the Colon and Rectum, London, UK

Principles and justification

Urethroscopy should be part of every cystoscopy in a male patient. There are those who also advocate that urethroscopy should immediately precede cystoscopy in female patients as well; certainly, there are no disadvantages to this. There are many advantages to a preliminary urethroscopy in male patients. The possibility of damaging the urethra is minimized by inserting an endoscope under direct vision.

Operations

RIGID CYSTOURETHROSCOPY

In women, the patient may be in either the lithotomy position or lying supine with the legs frogged. In men it is always easier and safer to perform a cystoscopy if the patient is in the lithotomy position.

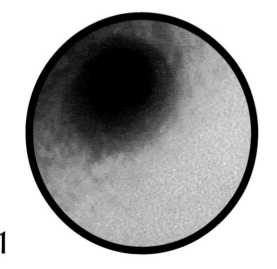

1 In male patients the penis is grasped as for catheterization, cleaned and a well-lubricated cystoscope with a 30° telescope is passed under vision down the urethra. The surgeon should be standing.

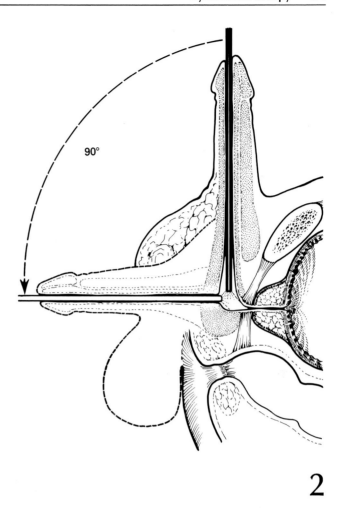

2

2 The cystoscope is advanced under vision until the bulbar urethra where the lumen will disappear. Keeping the tip of the cystoscope still, the surgeon's eye should move downwards through 90° while he assumes a sitting position. The tip of the cystoscope remains stationary.

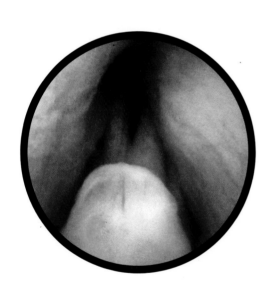

3

3 When the urethral lumen reappears the cystoscope may be safely advanced further, bringing into view the verumontanum, the prostatic urethra and the bladder neck.

The bladder should be emptied. With the wide-angle view of a 30° telescope it is possible to inspect the whole of the interior of the bladder. The irrigation is turned on and while the bladder is filling a quick inspection is made in each of the four quadrants. It is particularly helpful to be able to look at the anterior bladder wall during bladder filling.

When the bladder has been filled with 300–400 ml of irrigant a more detailed inspection is undertaken. Starting at the bladder neck at the 6 o'clock position, the cystoscope is passed as far as the posterior bladder wall during which the ureteric orifice will come into view.

The cystoscope is turned through 90° and the right lateral bladder wall is inspected from the bladder neck to the posterior bladder wall. The process is repeated at 12 o'clock and 3 o'clock. The ureteric orifices should be identified on each side.

FLEXIBLE CYSTOURETHROSCOPY

The availability of flexible cystoscopes has revolution-ized urological practice, allowing many diagnostic cystoscopies and check cystoscopies performed as part of the follow-up for bladder carcinoma to be performed under local anaesthesia on an outpatient basis.

The patient is asked to empty the bladder before the examination. The urethra is then cleaned as for a rigid cystoscopy and local anaesthetic jelly is instilled into the urethra and allowed to remain for 10 min to maximize its effect.

Under direct vision the urethra is inspected from distally to proximally. When the distal sphincter area in the male patient is reached the patient is asked to try to pass urine. This will have the effect of relaxing the sphincter and allowing more comfortable passage of the cystoscope through into the bladder.

A very thorough view of the bladder can be obtained by moving the flexible tip of the cystoscope.

Small cup biopsy forceps are available with which mucosal biopsies may be taken. Small bladder tumour recurrences can be coagulated using either bipolar diathermy or some form of neodymium laser.

Postoperative care

There should be no need for prophylactic antibiotics unless a urine infection has occurred in the recent past. The male and female urethra should be left well lubricated with anaesthetic jelly to minimize postopera-tive discomfort.

Complications

If a cystourethroscopy is correctly performed there is very little chance of causing damage. Perforation of the bladder, usually intraperitoneally, can occur and must be closed formally at laparostomy.

The incidence of urinary tract infections should be less than 3%.

Urethral dilatation

H. N. Whitfield MA, MChir, FRCS
Consultant Urologist, St Bartholomew's Hospital and St Mark's Hospital for Diseases of the Colon and Rectum, London, UK

History

There is evidence that urethral dilatation was performed in very primitive cultures using instruments fashioned from wood, ivory, elephant hairs, etc. In the 19th century de Guyon used filiform bougies. At the same time metal dilators, both straight and curved, were introduced by Ducamp. Urethral stricture formation was very common because of untreated venereal diseases. During the 19th century a variety of modifications to dilating instruments was developed.

Principles and justification

Indications

In women, particularly after the menopause, a urethral stenosis can occur which causes incomplete bladder emptying and provokes urinary infections. Such patients benefit from urethral dilatation or urethrotomy.

In men, urethral dilatation is now the treatment of choice for urethral strictures only in those patients who do not respond to an optical urethrotomy and in whom formal urethroplasty is contraindicated on the grounds of a general medical condition or is refused.

Operation

In female patients, straight dilators should be used progressively up to a size of 30 Fr. Care should be taken to dilate the full length of the urethra. The use of dilators which are not more than 10 cm long ensures that bladder perforation does not occur.

In male patients, dilatation can be difficult and may also provoke complications.

1a, b A meatal or submeatal stricture may be dilated safely with straight dilators. Strictures situated more proximally are treated using a curved sound such as a Clutton's or Liston's sound.

The urethra is well lubricated with local anaesthetic jelly. The tip of the dilator is then directed ventrally and the instrument is allowed to slide into the urethra under its own weight. When the tip of the dilator is at the level of the bulbar urethra the instrument should be rotated through 180° so that the tip is positioned to follow the direction of the urethra. The shaft of the penis is gently lowered through 90° while maintaining gentle pressure on the handle of the dilator to encourage onward progression.

The patient may often be able to tell if the dilator is being directed towards a false passage. When both the patient and the surgeon are confident that the dilator is within the bladder, confirmation can be obtained by rotating the handle of the instrument through 90° either side of 12 o'clock, which will have the effect of rotating the tip of the instrument from 9 o'clock, through 12 o'clock, to 3 o'clock within the bladder.

Postoperative care

A urethral catheter should not be necessary. Bleeding may occur but is seldom sufficient to provoke retention. The patient should be encouraged to drink a lot of fluid.

Complications

Bleeding may arise, and if this provokes clot retention a urethral catheter must be inserted. Septicaemia can occur even though prophylactic antibiotics have been administered.

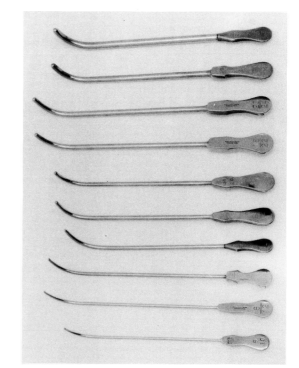

1a

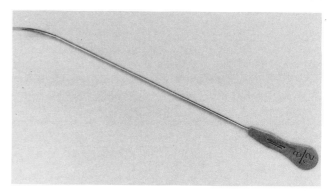

1b

Urethrotomy

H. N. Whitfield MA, MChir, FRCS
Consultant Urologist, St Bartholomew's Hospital and St Mark's Hospital for Diseases of the Colon and Rectum, London, UK

History

The instruments for urethrotomy, which were first described several centuries ago, provide evidence that urethral strictures in men have been a clinical problem for many years. Before antibiotics were available, gonococcal urethral strictures were common. Management consisted of either urethral dilatation or blind urethrotomy. The endoscopic management of urethral strictures has now changed, because a urethrotomy may be performed under vision. The underlying principle remains the same.

Instruments for dilating the urethra provided the impetus for the development of other methods for treating urethral strictures, one of the most common pathologies encountered in the urinary tract in the 19th and 20th centuries. The first urethrotome was designed by Oribase in about 368 AD. In 1878 Otis demonstrated his instrument, which has remained part of the urological armamentarium ever since. The first optical urethrotome was described by Desormeaux, but his instrument was used very little because there was no irrigation and bleeding obscured vision.

1 It was in 1974 that Sachse described the optical urethrotome that has been widely adopted since that time[1]. Strictures at any site in the urethra may be managed with this instrument.

The instrument has an oval circumference of 21 Fr. The working element is designed so that the cold knife remains within the sheath at rest and is then protruded from within the sheath by deflection of the thumb piece of the working element. A forward 0° telescope is used. The sheath incorporates an instrument channel, down which a flexible guidewire or ureteric catheter can be passed. A half-sheath can be attached to the instrument, so that following negotiation of the stricture a urethral catheter can be inserted without difficulty.

Principles and justification

Indications

In the male, a urethrotomy may be performed using a blind Otis urethrotome prophylactically, to prevent urethral strictures following transurethral resection of the prostate. The effectiveness of this procedure has been demonstrated by some authors[2, 3]. The procedure is only performed, however, after a preliminary cystourethroscopy has excluded any urethral pathology.

Strictures of almost any length, site and cause may be treated by an optical urethrotomy. There is evidence, however, that those that respond best are the short single strictures. These are usually located in the bulbar or membranous urethra. More extensive penile or bulbar strictures are better treated by open reconstructive surgery, as urethrotomy is associated with disappointing success rates[4].

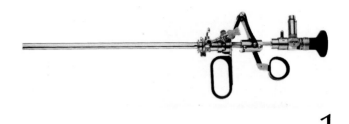

1

Preoperative

A prophylactic antibiotic should be administered before optical urethrotomy if there is a pre-existing urinary infection.

Operation

OTIS URETHROTOMY

For a blind urethrotomy using the Otis urethrotome, the well-lubricated instrument should be passed either as far as the bulbar urethra or, if preferred, into the bladder. The blades are then opened to the required degree to enable the knife of the instrument to cut the urethra to a calibre sufficiently large to accommodate the subsequent operating instrument without friction. In practice, if a transurethral prostatectomy is to be performed using a 24-Fr operating sheath, a urethrotomy can be performed safely at 26 Fr.

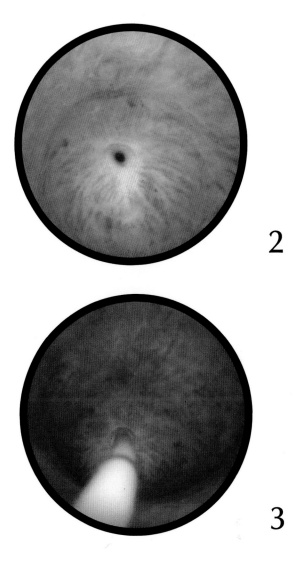

2

3

OPTICAL URETHROTOMY

2, 3 With the patient in the lithotomy position, the penis is cleaned and the instrument inserted under vision. When the urethral stricture is encountered, a guidewire or ureteric catheter should be inserted through the stricture and into the bladder.

This ensures that the subsequent urethrotomy is opening up the urethra and not creating a false passage.

4 The knife blade is protruded from the end of the sheath under vision alongside the guidewire, and the urethra is divided in the 12 o'clock position.

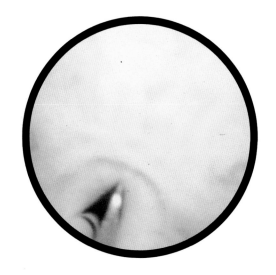

4

5–7 Cuts are made progressively more deeply until the lumen of the urethra is large enough to accommodate the sheath of the instrument.

Postoperative care

A urethral catheter is required for 24 h after Otis urethrotomy or optical urethrotomy to tamponade any bleeding that may occur from the corpus spongiosum.

Some surgeons advocate the use of hydrocortisone jelly installations in an attempt to reduce scar formation during healing after optical urethrotomy. Autodilatation of the urethra has been recommended by others. This is achieved by interrupting the urinary stream during micturition by pinching off the urethra close to the meatus. Alternatively, regular intermittent self-catheterization can be performed to achieve the same result.

Complications

Excessive bleeding following Otis urethrotomy can arise on occasions. This is best managed by inserting a urethral catheter, and the bleeding will usually stop spontaneously. If the instrument is inserted carelessly the tip may form a false passage in the urethra.

Some bleeding always occurs after optical urethrotomy, but on occasions can be very severe and require transfusion. Management consists of retaining a urethral catheter as a method of tamponading the bleeding. Despite adequate antibiotic prophylaxis, patients can develop septicaemia, particularly if there is a pre-existing urinary tract infection.

Outcome

About 85% of short urethral strictures in the male can be managed successfully by optical urethrotomy. Of the remaining 15%, a significant proportion will respond to a second urethrotomy. Thereafter, subsequent urethrotomies have progressively less chance of providing a long-term solution.

References

1. Sachse H. Zur Behandlung der Harnröhrenstriktur: die transurethrale Schlitzung unter Sicht mit scharfem Schnitt. *Fortschr Med* 1974; 92: 12–15.

2. Bailey MJ, Shearer RJ. The role of internal urethrotomy in the prevention of urethral stricture following transurethral resection of prostate. *Br J Urol* 1979; 51: 28–31.

3. Schultz A, Bay-Nielsen H, Bilde T, Christiansen L, Mikkelsen AM, Steven K. Prevention of urethral stricture formation after transurethral resection of the prostate: a controlled randomized study of Otis urethrotomy versus urethral dilatation and the use of the polytetrafluoroethylene coated versus the uninsulated metal sheath. *J Urol* 1989; 141: 73–5.

4. Sandozi S, Ghazali S. Sachse optical urethrotomy, a modified technique: 6 years of experience. *J Urol* 1988; 140: 968–9.

Sphincterotomy

H. N. Whitfield MA, MChir, FRCS
Consultant Urologist, St Bartholomew's Hospital and St Mark's Hospital for Diseases of the Colon and Rectum, London, UK

Principles and justification

This operation is most commonly performed for male patients who have a neuropathic bladder disorder which results in a combination of urinary incontinence and incomplete bladder emptying. It is likely that such patients will already have undergone bladder neck resection to ablate the bladder neck sphincter mechanism. If they are to be managed with a condom urinal it is essential that bladder emptying should be complete to reduce the chances of urinary infection and to avoid upper urinary tract obstruction.

Preoperative

A prophylactic antibiotic is esential since all these patients are likely to harbour a urinary pathogen.

Operation

Using the knife electrode in a resectoscope, the urethra is divided at 12 o'clock from the verumontanum distally for a distance of 2–3 cm. It is essential to incise through the urethral wall into the tissue of the corpus spongiosum. This will inevitably result in bleeding. Some authors advocate making incisions at 12 o'clock and 6 o'clock.

Postoperative care

A urethral catheter is necessary for 24–48 h.

Complications

Bleeding may be severe. Urinary infection and septicaemia can arise. It may be difficult to ablate the distal sphincter with this procedure as evidenced by the continuing presence of a residual urine volume. A further sphincterotomy is then required.

Illustrations by Peter Cox

Posterior urethral valves

Ian A. Aaronson MA, FRCS
Professor of Urology and Pediatrics and Director of Pediatric Urology, Medical University of South Carolina, Charleston, South Carolina, USA

Principles and justification

1 A posterior urethral valve is a single structure that takes origin from the inferior margin of the verumontanum. Although its embryology is uncertain, it lies in the position of the infracollicular folds, which can often be discerned in the normal posterior urethra running downwards from the verumontanum towards the bulb on either side of the midline.

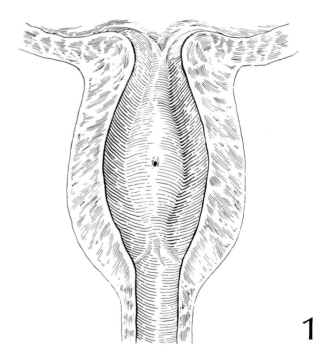

1

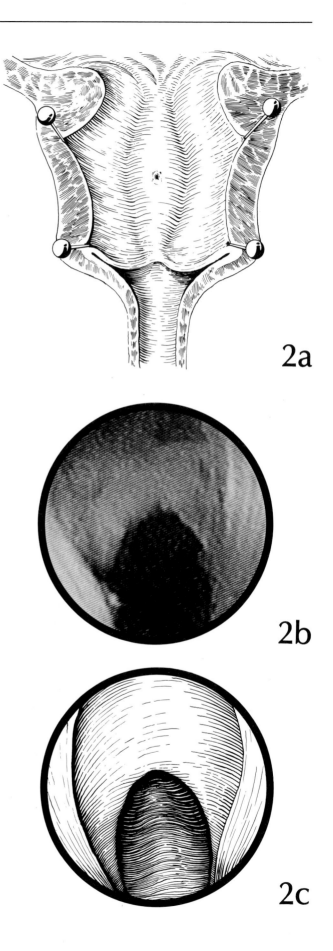

2a–c When exposed at autopsy through the anterior urethral wall, a posterior urethral valve appears as two separate leaflets, but on endoscopy these are seen to fuse anteriorly to form a curtain where most of the obstruction occurs.

Most valves are thin filmy structures that balloon downwards during voiding, but a few are thicker and more rigid, forming a transverse obstruction in the mid-posterior urethra. As all true valves originate from the inferior aspect of the verumontanum, Young's classification should be regarded as only of historic interest.

Minor degrees of valve are sometimes encountered, in which the two leaflets blend with the lateral urethral wall. They are more properly regarded as prominent infracollicular folds. It is unlikely that they ever cause symptoms or obstruction, and they do not require treatment.

Above the valve, back pressure effects are nearly always present; these are a widely dilated posterior urethra, a thick-walled and usually trabeculated bladder, widely dilated tortuous ureters and bilateral symmetrical hydronephrosis. Vesicoureteric reflux is common and often associated with a varying degree of dysplasia of the affected kidney.

The bladder neck is always thickened as part of detrusor hypertrophy, but this hardly ever causes obstruction or requires treatment.

Nowadays, the diagnosis is usually made either before birth as a result of antenatal ultrasonography, or immediately afterwards because of a persistently palpable bladder. Urinary ascites is an occasional presentation in the first weeks of life.

Infants in whom the diagnosis has been missed usually present with urinary infection and acute-on-chronic renal failure. This is generally accompanied by hyperkalaemia and a severe metabolic acidosis, which may lead to respiratory arrest. Water and sodium balance are often also profoundly disturbed. Septicaemia is common and may be complicated by a consumptive coagulopathy. Older boys may also present with urinary infection, but often the main complaint is of a poor stream with straining or urinary incontinence.

The diagnosis will usually be suspected on clinical grounds and will be supported by the ultrasonographic findings of a widened posterior urethra, distended bladder, and dilated upper urinary tract.

Preoperative

On suspicion of the diagnosis, an 8-Fr plastic infant feeding tube should be passed transurethrally and secured for continuous bladder drainage. Self-retaining catheters should be avoided, as the hypertrophied bladder tends to clamp down around the balloon and obstruct the ureters.

It is essential that the bladder drains well, and failure to do so is usually because the catheter has curled up in the dilated posterior urethra. Withdrawing the catheter for a few centimetres and repassing it with a finger in the rectum will usually ensure its passage through the hypertrophied bladder neck. Persistent difficulty can usually be resolved by injecting a few millilitres of contrast medium through the catheter and manipulating it under fluoroscopic control.

A full blood count including platelets, plasma electrolytes, creatinine and acid–base status should be determined, and severe derangements, particularly hyperkalaemia or a severe metabolic acidosis, should be corrected as a matter of urgency. An assessment should also be made of the infant's state of hydration. In difficult cases, the aid of a paediatric nephrologist should be sought.

When the urine appears to be infected, both a blood sample and a urine sample should be sent for culture, following which ampicillin and an aminoglycoside or a third-generation cephalosporin should be started intravenously. When septicaemia is suspected, blood coagulation studies should also be carried out.

All infants with any respiratory distress should undergo chest radiography to exclude a pneumothorax secondary to pulmonary hypoplasia.

In most cases the above actions will result in a rapid improvement in the infant's metabolic state and general condition. Those infants who remain in a toxic state or whose plasma creatinine does not begin to fall within 24 h despite correction of other metabolic abnormalities should be considered for percutaneous drainage of both kidneys.

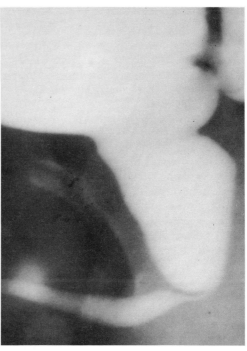

3a

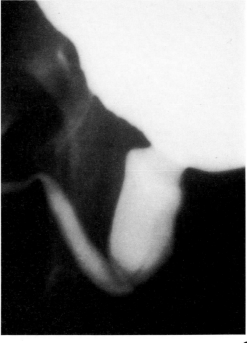

3b

3a, b The presence of a posterior urethral valve should be confirmed by micturating cysto-urethrography, but this should be delayed until urinary infection has been brought completely under control and metabolic disturbances have been corrected.

A voiding film during full micturition is necessary to demonstrate the valve, which appears like a sail billowing out before the stream. Distal to this a thin trickle can usually be seen emerging from the posterior margin of the obstruction (*Illustration 3a*). Dilatation of the urethra proximal to the valve is essential to the diagnosis, and signs of bladder wall hypertrophy are usually also present. A very lax valve may occasionally prolapse down as far as the bulbar urethra (*Illustration 3b*). Here the posterior run-off may not be readily apparent, but the filling defect caused by the valve leaflets can usually be made out running down from the verumontanum.

4a–h

A variety of other conditions may masquerade as a posterior urethral valve on the cystogram, and failure to recognize them often leads to inappropriate treatment. Among these are prominent infracollicular folds, which can sometimes be made out on a good quality study in normal children (*Illustration 4a*).

Hesitant voiding in a normal baby may cause an abrupt change in calibre of the posterior urethra, while extrinsic compression by the pelvic floor may cause one or more concentric indentations in the urethral contour (*Illustration 4b*). Neither of these is associated with evidence of obstruction above the lesion, however, and both should be regarded as normal variants.

A neuropathic bladder may closely simulate a posterior urethral valve (*Illustration 4c*), but the thin stream below the obstruction will be seen emerging from the centre of the external urethral sphincter rather than from the posterior margin as seen with a valve. In such cases, the spine should be carefully examined and other evidence sought of a neurological deficit in the perineum or lower limbs.

A posterior urethral stricture may cause a similar appearance (*Illustration 4d*), but this will invariably be associated with a history of urethral or pelvic trauma.

The prune-belly syndrome may closely mimic a posterior urethral valve (*Illustration 4e*) but the correct diagnosis should be suspected from the appearance of the bladder, which lies horizontally and is invariably smooth walled, and the dog-leg configuration of the posterior urethra, which often bears a utriculus masculinus.

A distended, non-visualized ectopic ureter opening into the ejaculatory duct may distort and partially obstruct the posterior urethra and thus simulate a valve (*Illustration 4f*), while dilatation of the posterior urethra may also be caused by a prolapsed ectopic ureterocoele (*Illustration 4g*) or posterior urethral polyp (*Illustration 4h*). Careful examination of these films, however, will usually reveal a filling defect, leading to the correct diagnosis.

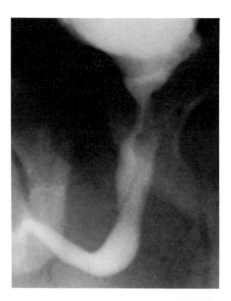

4a

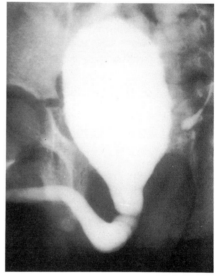

4b

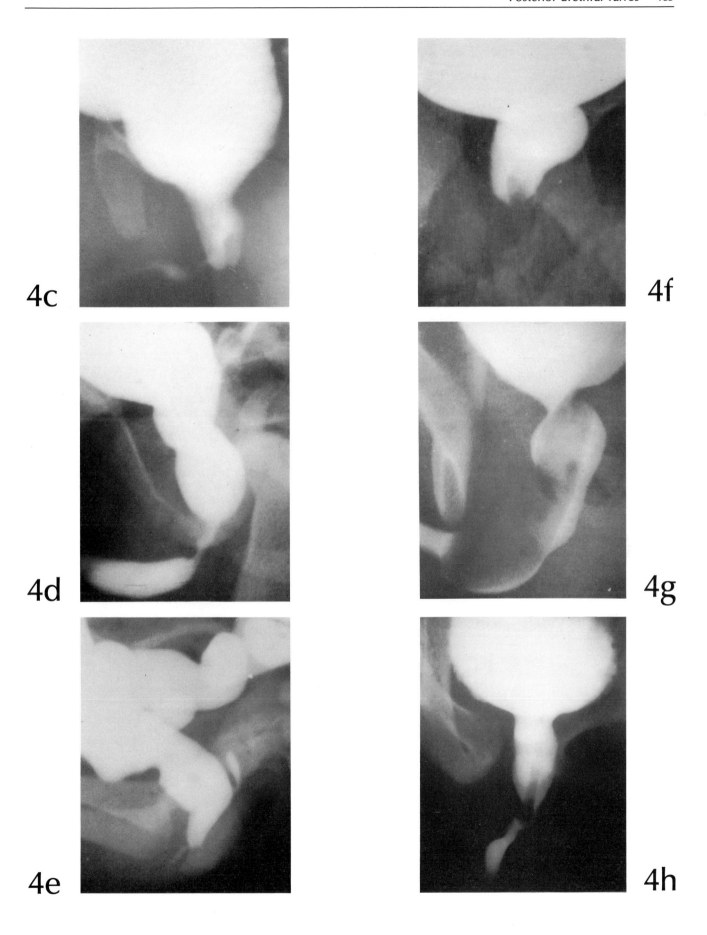

4c

4f

4d

4g

4e

4h

Operation

RESECTION IN FULL-TERM INFANTS AND CHILDREN

Under endotracheal anaesthesia, the intubated infant is placed supine with the buttocks brought well down to the end of the operating table. The legs should be well protected with cotton wool and fixed with crepe bandages, either to paediatric stirrups or in the frog-leg position, taking care to provide ample support to the thighs. The skin is prepared and drapes applied, taking care to exclude the anus from the operative field. Fixing the posterior towel to the perineal skin with three 4/0 nylon sutures will ensure that the anus does not become exposed during subsequent manipulations.

The calibre of the penile urethra should first be checked with a well-lubricated 10-Fr sound, which should be introduced only for 1–2 cm. If necessary, a meatotomy can be performed, but no attempt should be made to dilate the urethra. The diagnosis is then confirmed using a well-lubricated 9.5-Fr or 10-Fr cystoscope introduced under vision.

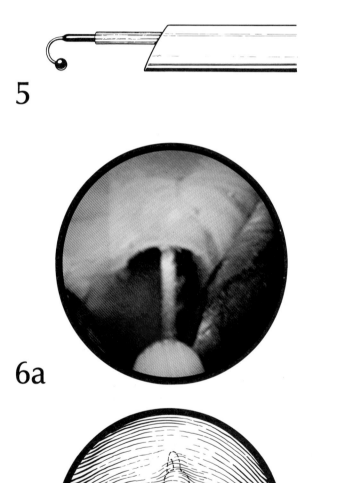

5

6a

6b

— Valve

Resectoscope
sheath

— Verumontanum

5 Resection of the valve is undertaken using a 10-Fr Storz resectoscope fitted with a hooked ball electrode.

The instrument is first assembled and the alignment of the working parts checked using the 0° telescope. The sheath is then dried and thoroughly coated with a water-soluble lubricant, and with its introducer in place is gently inserted through the meatus. The introducer is removed and the instrument reassembled and gently advanced under vision towards the bladder neck. It is often necessary to angle the eyepiece end of the instrument downwards to allow the beak to move anteriorly to pass through the bladder neck. Once in the bladder, the shape and position of the ureteric orifices are noted and the presence of any periureteric diverticulum recorded.

6a, b The instrument is rotated through 180°, and with the irrigation fluid flowing in under low pressure, it is progressively withdrawn. Once through the bladder neck, the ball is run down along the anterior wall of the posterior urethra until, just beyond the verumontanum, the valve will suddenly snap across the anterior portion of the field of view like a curtain. Further withdrawal of the instrument and manipulation of the trigger will cause the ball to engage the valve in the 12 o'clock position. A short burst of cutting current is then applied.

7a–d

The instrument is returned to the normal position and advanced under vision back into the bladder. It is again rotated 180° and withdrawn into the posterior urethra to engage the now partially disrupted valve in the 12 o'clock position, where it is further disrupted. This manoeuvre should be repeated until it is certain that the anterior portion of the valve has been completely ablated.

The instrument is again returned to the bladder and is rotated to engage residual valve tissue in the 10 o'clock, 2 o'clock, 8 o'clock and finally the 4 o'clock positions. Any remaining freely floating tags do not require treatment.

The resectoscope is removed and the presence of an unobstructed urethra confirmed by manual expression of the bladder. Finally, an 8-Fr feeding tube is passed, placing a double-gloved finger in the rectum if necessary to ensure that it is not curled up in the dilated posterior urethra. This is retained in place with a 4/0 nylon suture passed through the prepuce or glans and connected to a sealed drainage bag. The tube is removed after 48 h.

If any significant bleeding occurs, attempts at valve ablation should be immediately discontinued and the situation reassessed after 2–3 days of catheter drainage.

In older children a 13-Fr resectoscope may be used, employing a similar technique.

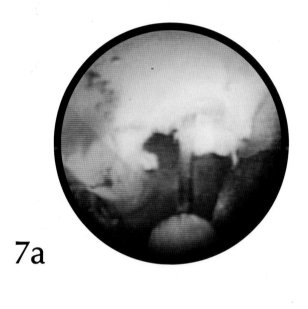

7a

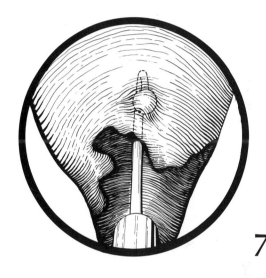

7b

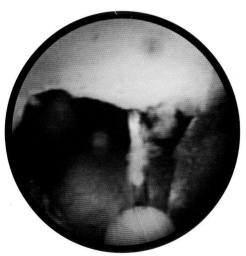

7c

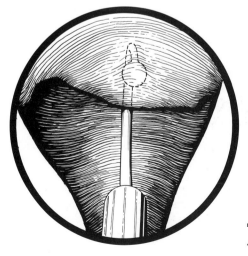

7d

RESECTION IN PRETERM INFANTS

It is inadvisable to attempt to pass a 10-Fr resectoscope in infants weighing less than 2.5 kg. For those between 2.0 and 2.5 kg, an 8-Fr feeding tube may be passed into the bladder and left connected to a drainage bag for a few days. This will often have the effect of gently dilating the urethra so that the 10-Fr resectoscope can be safely used.

In infants weighing less than 2.0 kg, one of several procedures may be employed.

The newly available 8-Fr operating cystoscope (Storz) can usually be introduced into the urethra in all but the smallest infants. A 3-Fr ureteric catheter is introduced through the working channel, and the exposed end of the metal stylet is used to coagulate the valve in a circumferential fashion.

The Whitaker hook electrode (Cambmac Instruments Ltd, Cambridge, UK) is a well-insulated and relatively atraumatic instrument that can be introduced into the posterior urethra under fluoroscopic control and withdrawn to engage the valve. A short burst of cutting current in the 12 o'clock, 9 o'clock and 3 o'clock positions will usually relieve the obstruction.

In antegrade endoscopic disruption, a good view of the valve is first obtained with a 10-Fr resectoscope introduced via the bladder neck through a formal cystotomy. The valve is then ablated by electrocautery using the ball electrode, beginning in the 12 o'clock position. The bladder is closed and drained by a catheter, which is left in place for 1 week.

Access to the valve by a 10-Fr resectoscope can usually be achieved via a perineal urethrotomy. The small calibre of the urethra and the friable nature of the urothelium, however, render the operation difficult in the newborn, and it may be complicated by bleeding, a stricture, a persistent urinary fistula, or a urethral diverticulum.

A Fogarty catheter can be passed into the bladder, where the balloon is inflated with 0.2–0.5 ml of water. It is then withdrawn until the balloon is felt to engage the valve. Disruption may be achieved by a further short sharp pull on the catheter. If undue resistance is encountered, however, the procedure should be discontinued to avoid possible avulsion of the urethra.

In very small babies, the bladder may be drained by a 5-Fr infant feeding tube for several weeks to allow growth to occur. Frequent monitoring of the urine is necessary, however, to ensure that it remains free of infection.

Vesicostomy is the best means of obtaining relief of obstruction in small infants when specialized instruments are not available or when unexpected difficulties arise during attempted endoscopic ablation.

ADDITIONAL SURGERY

This may be indicated when there is a persistently raised plasma creatinine or persistent unilateral reflux.

Following relief of the urethral obstruction, correction of metabolic derangements and eradication of infection, the plasma creatinine will rapidly fall to within the normal range for the patient's age in most infants. When it remains elevated, partial obstruction of the dilated flaccid ureters as they pass through the hypertrophied bladder wall must be considered. In most cases this phenomenon is transient, and provided that the infant remains well and the plasma creatinine is showing some improvement, an expectant policy may be adopted. In severe cases, a Whitaker test should be carried out and, if positive, Sober Y cutaneous ureterostomies should be performed[1]. Alternatively, the ureters may be remodelled and reimplanted, but the operation is exacting and in inexperienced hands complications are common.

In cases of persistent unilateral reflux, renal scanning using ^{99m}Tc-DMSA (dimercaptosuccinic acid) will usually show that the kidney on the affected side has negligible function. Nephroureterectomy is carried out, preferably through two incisions, to ensure safe ligation of the ureteric stump flush with the bladder.

Postoperative care

At 48 h, a prophylactic antibiotic, usually trimethoprim–sulphamethoxozole, is commenced and given for 1 month to guard against infection in the healing posterior urethra. This is continued for 6 months in those infants in whom cystography reveals the presence of vesicoureteric reflux. Sodium bicarbonate supplements are also often necessary to correct a persistent metabolic acidosis, and these may need to be continued for 1 year or more. Polyuria is also common, and the parents should be advised to give supplementary clear feeds early in the event of a diarrhoeal illness.

At 3 months, the glomerular filtration rate of each kidney is measured by the slope clearance method using ^{99m}Tc-DTPA (diethylenetriaminepenta-acetate), and intravenous urography is carried out. Both of these will serve as a baseline for any subsequent studies. A blood sample is also taken to check the plasma creatinine, electrolytes and acid–base status.

8 At 6 months, micturating cystourethrography is repeated to confirm adequate resection of the valve and the absence of any stricture of the urethra, and to determine whether vesicoureteric reflux is still present. In about one-third of cases it will be found to have disappeared. When reflux is persistent and unilateral, renal scanning using ^{99m}Tc-DMSA is carried out to determine the contribution of the refluxing kidney to total renal function.

All infants and those older children with impaired renal function at presentation will require close supervision until adult life is reached. A progressive rise in plasma creatinine is often seen during childhood, and in the most severe cases renal transplantation may be required before puberty. Persistent urinary incontinence is an indication for cystometrography. Bladders showing severe hyper-reflexia or very poor compliance may require augmentation before transplantation.

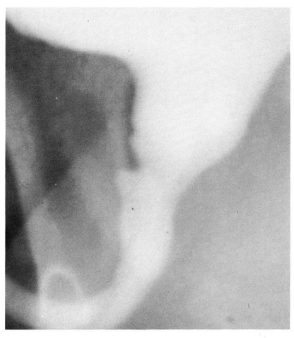

8

Further reading

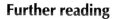

Aaronson IA. Posterior urethral valve: a review of 120 cases. *S Afr Med J* 1984; 65: 418–22.

Crombleholme TM, Harrison MR, Langer JC *et al*. Early experience with open fetal surgery for congenital hydronephrosis. *J Pediatr Surg* 1988; 23: 1114–21.

Parkhouse HF, Barratt TM, Dillon MJ *et al*. Long term outcome of boys with posterior urethral valves. *Br J Urol* 1988; 62: 59–62.

Reference

1. Rickwood AMK. Ureterostomy. In: Whitfield HN, ed. *Rob and Smith's Operative Surgery. Genitourinary Surgery*. 5th edn. Vol. 2. pp. 821–31.

Urethral stents

Euan Milroy FRCS
Consultant Urologist, The Middlesex Hospital, London, UK

History

The treatments presently used for urethral strictures all have their limitations, and most urologists would agree that despite the many techniques available there are still a number of patients with recurrent and difficult strictures for whom satisfactory alternative treatments would be useful. It was for this reason that the author started using the Urolume Wallstent (American Medical Systems, Minneapolis, Minnesota, USA) for the treatment of recurrent strictures of the bulbar urethra[1]. Recently other manufacturers have become interested in endoscopic stenting for urethral strictures, but at present the Urolume stent is the only one with which extensive experience has been gained and which is commercially available.

This stent was first invented by Hans Wallsten for endovascular insertion into the arterial system, with the aim of preventing restenosis after transluminal angioplasty. In the vascular tree the stent was found to become covered with endothelium, and this device is still being used with considerable success[2].

Urolume stent

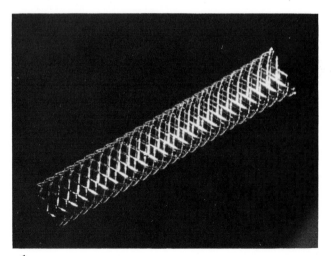

1

1 The Urolume Wallstent is a woven tubular mesh of fine corrosion-resistant superalloy wire. The stent can be made in any length and diameter, but at the present time is only available for urethral use in lengths of 20 mm and 30 mm, both of which are 14 mm in diameter. It is important to note that these measurements refer to the stent in its unconstrained state. When implanted into the urethra, the stent will be smaller in diameter and correspondingly longer. When released from its delivery system the stent springs open and the radial force of the mesh holds it against the wall of the previously dilated urethral stricture, allowing urothelium to grow over the implanted material whilst holding open the strictured area[3, 4].

The author has also used the same stent to relieve prostate obstruction[5] – for this indication a greater range of lengths and diameters is now available – and also to hold open the dyssynergic urethral sphincter as an alternative to sphincterotomy in patients with traumatic tetraplegia and sphincter dyssynergia[6]. The finding that this stent will hold open strictures while becoming covered with epithelium has encouraged its use in a number of strictures in the biliary system and the trachea. Limited experience is also being gained with smaller diameter stents in ureteric obstruction.

Principles and justification

Indications

2a, b The Urolume stent should, in general, be used only for the treatment of recurrent strictures of the bulbar urethra, between the distal urethral sphincter mechanism and the penoscrotal junction. Inserting the stent into a stricture involving the sphincter mechanism may be a satisfactory treatment for the stricture but will, of course, compromise continence. Continence in this case may be maintained by a competent bladder neck or by the subsequent insertion of an artificial urinary sphincter. The author has used this latter combination with success in a number of cases, but it does require special expertise and is not recommended. Using the stent in the pendulous penile urethra may cause pain and distortion during erection. The pain will usually settle in time, but the stent should not be used downstream of the penoscrotal junction if the patient is sexually active.

Because long-term experience of the stent is limited, it should not be used as the first treatment of any urethral stricture. It is well known that a number of strictures will be cured by a single dilatation or urethrotomy, and it would be unwise to implant one of these devices until the stricture has been found to recur after one or two urethrotomies or dilatations. It should be noted, however, that repeated treatment will encourage the development of further fibrosis, which may in fact jeopardize the long-term result of the stent. A number of patients have been seen who have grown fibrous tissue into the lumen of the stent, causing recurrent obstruction. This has occurred particularly after complete rupture of the bulbar or membranous urethra resulting in dense stricture formation, and the Urolume stent should therefore not be used in traumatic strictures. These patients are very satisfactorily treated with a single-stage anastomotic urethroplasty. The other group of patients who tend to develop increased fibrosis within the lumen of the stent are those whose urethral strictures have recurred following inlay urethroplasty procedures, presumably because of the introduction of squamous epithelium, which covers the stent less satisfactorily, into an already very scarred area. This problem of stent fibrosis has also been noted in a few patients with very long histories of multiple previous treatments.

In the present state of experience, this stent should not be used in strictures longer than 3–4 cm because of the length of implanted material which would then encroach on the sphincter or penile urethra and, except in the most exceptional circumstances, it should not be used in those younger than 30 years of age until long-term results become available. It would also be inappropriate to use any permanently implanted device

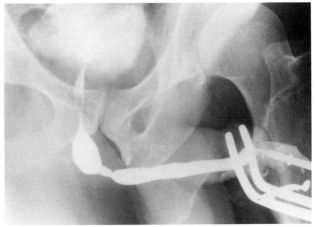

2a

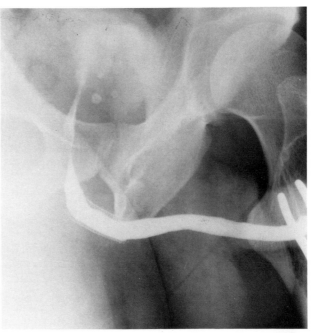

2b

of this sort in a chronically infected urethral stricture with periurethral abscess formation and fistulae.

Despite these warnings and limitations, the stent remains an excellent and highly successful treatment for the most common type of stricture now found in most urological practices, i.e. iatrogenic stricture of the bulbar urethra following catheterization or instrumentation, or the short infective stricture recurring after one or two urethrotomies or dilatations.

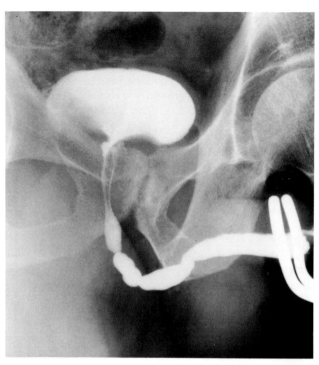

3a

Preoperative

$3a, b$ A urethrogram is essential before deciding on whether the stricture is suitable for this treatment. If possible both a retrograde and an antegrade (or voiding) study should be performed, to outline adequately both the upper and lower limits of the stricture and to ensure that the stricture is within an area suitable for stenting. It is important that the study is carried out by an experienced radiologist or urologist with adequate distension (but not over-distension) of the urethra. A urine flow rate is a useful measure of the degree of obstruction, though it is important to remember that the flow rate depends not only on urethral resistance but also on bladder pressure. By increasing bladder pressure a reasonable flow rate may be maintained despite considerable narrowing of the urethra. This is particularly important to remember when assessing the postoperative results of treating urethral strictures. A urethrogram and endoscopy is as important as a measurement of urine flow rate.

A urine culture is essential before stent insertion. If a urinary infection is present it should be treated vigorously for at least 10 days before dilatation and stent insertion, and for 2 weeks after surgery. If the urine is sterile it is advisable to cover the stent insertion with a single dose of broad-spectrum antibiotic at the time of surgery.

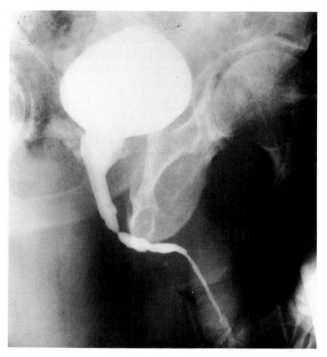

3b

Operation

The Urolume stent may be inserted under a general anaesthetic or, if it is known that the stricture will be easy to dilate or has been dilated recently, local urethral anaesthesia.

The stricture must first be dilated to allow the stent delivery system to be introduced into the urethra. It is probably safer to use filiform bougies with screw-on following dilators to reduce the risk of false passages and excess damage to the urethra. If the stricture is very tight or difficult to dilate, an endoscopic optical urethrotomy may be necessary. It is important not to cut too deeply into the wall of the urethra or there is a risk that the stent may be displaced outside the true line of the urethra. If urethrotomy is used it is therefore preferable to make three more superficial radial cuts in the urethra rather than one deep cut. If possible the urethra should be dilated to 30 Fr, but if the penile urethra is too small to accommodate this size of bougie, dilatation to 26 Fr or 28 Fr is sufficient.

After dilatation of the stricture a urethroscopy and cystoscopy should be carried out to make sure that the rest of the urethra is normal and to check on the position of the proximal end of the stricture in relation to the urethral sphincter. It is also important to exclude any bladder pathology. The length of damaged urethra should then be measured. This can be done using the preoperative urethrogram, but a check can also be made with a calibrated ureteric catheter after dilatation of the stricture.

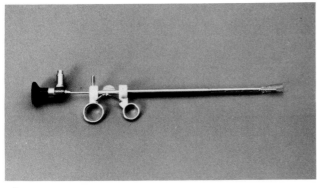

4a

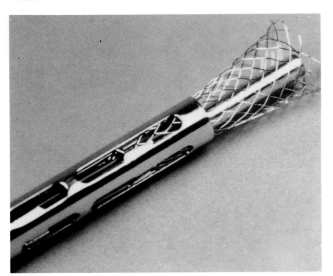

4b

4a, b The stent is supplied by the manufacturer loaded on its delivery system in a sterile pack. At the present time, stents of 2 and 3 cm in length are available for use in urethral strictures. When implanted into the urethra, an overlap of 0.5 cm should be allowed into normal urethra on each side of the stricture, and allowance must also be made for the fact that when the stent is inserted into a urethra of diameter smaller than 14 mm the length when implanted will be correspondingly longer.

The delivery system provided by the manufacturer is also supplied with a comprehensive instruction manual and it is important to study this carefully before using the device for the first time.

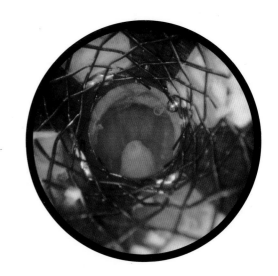

5

5 A standard 0° telescope is first introduced into the delivery system and a water or normal saline irrigating system is attached to the irrigation port. The delivery system can then be introduced through the external urethral meatus up the urethra under direct vision into the area of the previously dilated stricture. Once in position the first safety lock should be removed, allowing deployment of the stent. The inner end of the stent must be approximately 0.75 mm upstream of the end of the stricture in order to allow for some expansion and shortening of the stent during deployment.

6a, b The stent is deployed by pulling back the index finger towards the thumb which pulls back the outer sheath of the introducer from the stent. It is very important that only the index finger moves. The thumb must remain fixed in position otherwise the stent itself will tend to move (it may be easier to use two hands to work the mechanism rather than thumb and index finger). The stent is opened until the second lock is reached, at which point the position can be checked by sliding the telescope in and out of the delivery system. The most common mistake is to implant the upstream (bladder) end of the stent too close to the margin of the stricture itself. A 0.5-cm overlap must be allowed for.

If the position of the stent is judged to be correct the second lock is removed and the outer sheath pulled back to release the stent completely. If the position is not correct the index finger can be pushed forwards to advance the outer sheath over the stent. Once the stent is fully enclosed by the sheath it can then be repositioned in the urethra and deployed again as necessary. When the second lock has been removed and the stent fully deployed it is important to check that the stent has been fully released from the delivery system before the system is pulled out of the urethra. The simplest way to check this is to rotate gently the delivery system a few degrees whilst observing the outer end of the stent. If the stent is still attached gentle manoeuvring of the delivery system will release it without difficulty. The thumb should then be pulled back in order to retract the three stent clamps into the sheath before the delivery system is removed from the urethra. It is now a good idea to replace the second locking device as this will ensure that the stent clamps are fully retracted before moving the delivery system down the urethra.

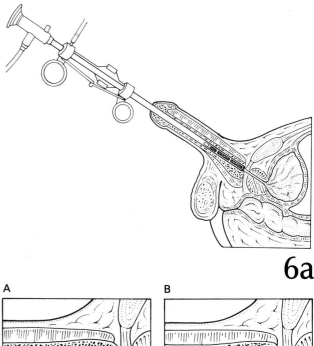

6a

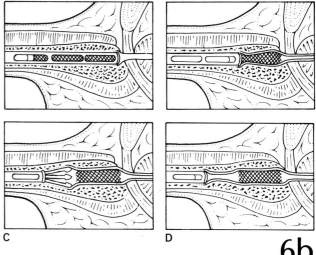

A

B

C

D

6b

7 If required the delivery instrument may be used to observe the stent itself, by advancing the system through the centre of the stent up into the bladder which may then be emptied before completing the procedure. Before this manoeuvre is carried out it is essential that the stent clamps are fully retracted and locked in position with the second locking device. Alternatively a 19-Fr cystoscope can be used to check the stent position after deployment, and to empty the bladder at the end of the procedure.

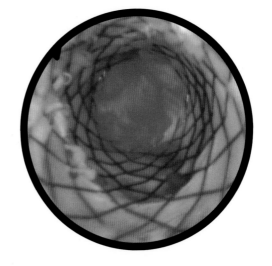

7

Postoperative care

8 It is important that no urethral catheter should be passed for the first 2–3 weeks after stent insertion. Very occasionally, particularly if a difficult optical urethrotomy has caused bleeding, the stent may fill with blood clots and the patient is unable to void. When the bladder is palpable a suprapubic catheter should be introduced using local anaesthesia. Normal voiding will be re-established in 24–48 h.

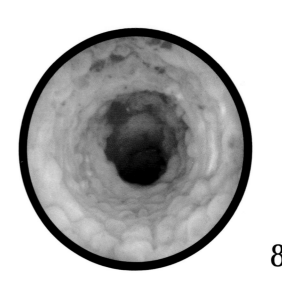

8

Patients are usually discharged the following day, though if the dilatation is not difficult they may return home as soon as they have demonstrated that they can pass urine without difficulty.

Patients should be warned that some initial discomfort in the perineum may be experienced, but that this will pass after 3–4 weeks. They should be cautioned to avoid cycling and horse-riding for a period of 1–2 months, and cyclists should then use a wide-base saddle to avoid pressure on the area of the stent. Occasional urethral bleeding may be seen for 1–2 weeks, and a few patients have noticed discomfort with erection and rather watery semen for the first 2–3 months, though this settles with time. Many patients, particularly those with 3-cm stents, will experience some post-micturition dribbling of urine which will be worse with any exertion. In the majority this problem will resolve spontaneously in the first 3–6 months, though about

15% of patients will continue to have a small amount of dribbling after this time. This is seldom of any serious significance and is usually easily managed with a little tissue or disposable 'mini-pad' inside the underclothes. This dribbling appears to come from the hyperplastic reaction to the stent during the first few months after insertion, and also from the small amount of urine that is held within the lumen of the epithelialized stent after the completion of micturition.

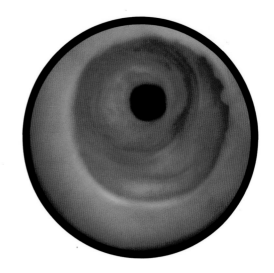

9 Patients should be followed with regular urine flow rate measurements and urethrograms every 6 months for the first 2–3 years, together with endoscopy, if there is any suggestion of problems with the device. The hyperplastic reaction seen in a number of patients can produce a most alarming appearance on the ascending urethrogram, but this will be found to settle in the majority of patients. The hyperplasia is particularly severe in patients whose strictures have followed a failed urethroplasty, and in these patients there is an increased incidence of subsequent fibrous tissue developing within the lumen of the stent.

The same problem has been seen in patients with traumatic complete rupture strictures, where the degree of intrastent fibrosis may completely block the stent. For this reason this device should not be used in traumatic strictures and should be used with great care in post-urethroplasty strictures. Patients should be warned about the possibility of restenosis, and although the fibrous tissue can easily be resected from within the stent, further surgical procedures may be necessary in such patients after this complication.

Until long-term results are available, the Urolume stent should be used with caution, but it certainly has a useful place in the treatment of bulbar urethral strictures that are not amenable to a simple anastomotic repair, or that have recurred after one or two dilatations or urethrotomies but have not yet developed a large amount of aggressive periurethral fibrous tissue.

9

References

1. Milroy EJG, Chapple CR, Cooper JE *et al*. A new treatment for urethral strictures. *Lancet* 1988; i: 1424–7.

2. Sigwart U, Puel J, Mirkovitch V, Joffre F, Kappenberger L. Intra-vascular stents to prevent occlusion and restenosis after transluminal angioplasty. *N Engl J Med* 1987; 316: 701–6.

3. Milroy EJG, Chapple C, Eldin A, Wallsten H. A new treatment for urethral strictures: a permanently implanted urethral stent. *J Urol* 1989; 141: 1120–2.

4. Sarramon JP, Joffre F, Rischmann P, Rousseau H, Eldin A, Wallsten H. Prosthèse endo-uréthrale 'Wallstent' dans les sténoses récidivant de l'urèthre. *Ann Urol* 1989; 23: 383–7.

5. Chapple CR, Milroy EJG, Rickards D. Permanently implanted urethral stent for prostatic obstruction in the unfit patient. *Br J Urol* 1990; 66: 58–65.

6. Shaw PJR, Milroy EJG, Timoney AG, Eldin A, Mitchell N. Permanent external striated sphincter stents in patients with spinal injuries. *Br J Urol* 1990; 66: 297–302.

Index